Caring for Prostate
Cancer Survivors

of related interest

Acupuncture and Cancer Survivorship
Recovery, Renewal, and Transformation
Beverley de Valois
Forewords by Jennifer A. Stone MSOM, LAc and Dr Catherine Zollman MBBS, MRCP, MRCGP
ISBN 978 1 91342 627 9
eISBN 978 1 91342 628 6

Yoga Therapy across the Cancer Care Continuum
Leigh Leibel and Anne Pitman
Foreword by Lorenzo Cohen
ISBN 978 1 91208 591 0
eISBN 978 1 91208 592 7

Adapting Yoga for People Living with Cancer
Jude Mills
Foreword by Charlotte Watts
ISBN 978 1 78775 650 2
eISBN 978 1 78775 651 9

Oncology Massage
An Integrative Approach to Cancer Care
Janet Penny and Rebecca Sturgeon
Foreword by Cal Cates
ISBN 978 1 91208 575 0
eISBN 978 1 91208 576 7

Aromatherapy, Massage and Relaxation in Cancer Care
An Integrative Resource for Practitioners
Edited by Ann Carter and Dr Peter A. Mackereth
ISBN 978 1 84819 281 2
eISBN 978 0 85701 228 9

CARING FOR PROSTATE CANCER SURVIVORS

A Biopsychosocial Approach in Physiotherapy and Oncology Practice

SAMANTHA HUGHES, MScPT

Foreword by Carolyn Vandyken
Illustrations by Adriano Renzi

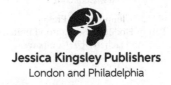

Jessica Kingsley Publishers
London and Philadelphia

First published in Great Britain in 2024 by Jessica Kingsley Publishers
Part of John Murray Press

1

The information contained in this book is not intended to replace the services
of trained medical professionals or to be a substitute for medical advice. You
are advised to consult a doctor on any matters relating to your health, and in
particular on any matters that may require diagnosis or medical attention.

A CIP catalogue record for this title is available from the
British Library and the Library of Congress

ISBN 978 1 83997 669 8
eISBN 978 1 83997 670 4

Printed and bound in the United States by Integrated Books International

Jessica Kingsley Publishers' policy is to use papers that are natural, renewable
and recyclable products and made from wood grown in sustainable
forests. The logging and manufacturing processes are expected to conform
to the environmental regulations of the country of origin.

Jessica Kingsley Publishers
Carmelite House
50 Victoria Embankment
London EC4Y 0DZ

www.jkp.com

John Murray Press
Part of Hodder & Stoughton Limited
An Hachette UK Company

This book is dedicated to the patients, mentors, researchers, and healthcare professionals who have inspired and supported me throughout my journey in prostate cancer care. To my patients, thank you for entrusting me with your care and for allowing me to be a part of your journey. You have taught me invaluable lessons and inspired me with your strength, humility, and resilience. To my mentors, thank you for guiding and shaping me into the healthcare professional I am today. Your wisdom, experience, and support have been instrumental in my growth and development. To researchers, thank you for your ongoing commitment to this field, and for the invaluable contributions in advancing our understanding of prostate cancer and treatments. And to all healthcare professionals working in prostate cancer care, thank you for your unwavering commitment and dedication to improving the lives of those affected by this disease. This book is a tribute to all of you, and I hope that it will serve as a source of inspiration and guidance to others in this field.

Contents

Part 1: Understanding Prostate Cancer Treatments and Effects

Part 2: The Biopsychosocial Approach in Caring for Prostate Cancer Survivors

Appendices

Foreword

Carolyn Vandyken

PROSTATE CANCER SURVIVORSHIP: BUILDING SELF-EFFICACY THROUGH A BIOPSYCHOSOCIAL LENS

As a physiotherapist for the past 37 years, I have had the opportunity to witness the important transition within physiotherapy practice from a biomechanical, tissue-focused approach to a humanistic, biopsychosocial approach. As clinicians, the person in front of us is always complex and "messy," which is the nature of our human lives, especially when injury or illness enters the picture.

My practice dramatically changed 15 years ago when I took a brilliant course from one of our physiotherapy leaders in Canada, Debbie Patterson. I have never looked back. My outcomes improved dramatically, and it took the pressure off me to "fix" my patients. This humanistic, biopsychosocial approach puts the patient in the "driver's seat" and requires collaboration between the patient and their healthcare providers.

Sam Hughes and I crossed paths in a similar way to Debbie and myself, except the roles were reversed. Sam listened to me speak at a pelvic pain conference, and she had her own "ah-ha" moment. Sam has taken several courses from me on this patient-centered, compassion-based, and culturally sensitive approach, embracing it to the fullest. Sam cares deeply for her patients, particularly for her male pelvic health patients. Sam has an impressive track record of instituting many programs over the years to help prostate cancer survivors' live life to the fullest.

This passion for both her patients and a biopsychosocial approach were the underlying reasons for Sam to write this book. Too many patients are still undergoing prostate cancer rehabilitation from a purely biomechanical, pelvic-floor-muscle training approach.

There are many similarities between persistent pain care, cancer care, and the approach that Sam describes in detail in this book, namely a biopsychosocial, whole-person approach. In rehabilitation, personalized persistent pain care from a biopsychosocial perspective has been called upon to replace outdated biomechanical and biomedical beliefs. In cancer care, a personalized, biopsychosocial plan is equally important, not only for survival, but for living well after medical care has been delivered. Living well after a cancer diagnosis does not stop at the completion of medical intervention.

The complexities of this approach include addressing the physical, psychological, and social needs of the individual patient with the goal of building self-efficacy and resiliency. Indeed, self-efficacy may be the cornerstone to living well with prostate cancer and beyond. As Mahatma Gandhi put it, "If I have the belief that I can 'do it', I shall surely acquire the capacity to 'do it' even if I may not have it at the beginning."[1] This wasn't just an inspirational soundbite: it was good psychology. Our faith in our own abilities to succeed plays a major role in whether we do so. Gandhi's philosophy is, to some extent, a self-fulfilling prophecy.

As clinicians, do we build our patient's capacity to "do it" and live well in every domain of life? Prostate cancer impacts not only one's physical self, but also each man's psychological state, behavior, and motivation, which directly impacts self-efficacy. This timely and well-written book will help clinicians and patients alike to develop a strong sense of self-efficacy when dealing with prostate cancer and the implications of both treatment and survivorship.

To build self-efficacy, a biopsychosocial approach to recovery and resiliency is built on several key factors that are distilled in this book. The first is to view challenging problems as tasks to be mastered, for example, incontinence and loss of sexual function. Breaking down the patient's experiences into the physical, psychological, and social implications will help him to identify the issues in each domain and address them accordingly.

Second, the goal is to deeply develop patients' interest in their rehabilitation activities. Too often, patients are working on the clinician's "goals" in therapy, not their own. Lack of adherence in rehabilitation is often rooted in a failure to set goals for recovery that bring value and joy to the patient. When non-compliance enters the therapy room, question yourself as the clinician, not the patient. What are you missing? What are their goals? Do these align with your goals?

The third step in building self-efficacy is to help patients form a strong sense of commitment to their goals. Too many clinicians are still uncomfortable talking to patients about their sexual goals. Patients often give up on recovering some level of sexual intimacy and it is our job to build excitement

---

1   Gandhi (1942)

and expectancy that intimacy can be recovered. There is an entire chapter in this book dedicated to helping clinicians and patients bridge this gap.

The fourth skill that clinicians need to create stronger self-efficacy is to help patients recover quickly from setbacks and disappointment. Injustice around the diagnosis of cancer ("why me?"), and the implication of functional loss in the realm of sexual health, need to be addressed within an interdisciplinary team, so that survivors don't overly focus on personal failings and negative outcomes. This skill starts with measuring injustice (utilizing the Injustice Experience Questionnaire) so that non-mental-health clinicians can help to identify anger and injustice in their patient's stories. It is by identifying these components of a patient's story that a true comprehensive, interdisciplinary approach is born.

Sam has done an excellent job of weaving the importance of survivorship into living well. This book will guide patients towards making informed choices about acute care, as well as engaging with appropriate, ongoing rehabilitation support to build self-efficacy and the belief that life can be "lived well" after a prostate cancer diagnosis.

Carolyn Vandyken, registered physiotherapist
Owner, Reframe Rehab, biopsychosocial-focused education

REFERENCE

Gandhi, M. (1942). *Non-Violence in Peace and War, 1st edition*. Ahmedabad, India: Navajivan Publishing House.

Acknowledgments

I would like to express my deep appreciation for the support and encouragement of the many people in my life who have made it possible for me to write this book. I am immensely grateful to my friend and colleague, Shelly Prosko, who introduced me to Jessica Kingsley Publishers and provided invaluable insights into compassionate care. I am also thankful for the health professionals and prostate cancer survivors who generously shared their time and knowledge to make this book more personable and informative, including Joy Egilson and Paul Griggs from the Prostate Cancer Supportive Care Program in Vancouver, and Robert Orr from Life 360 Innovations. I couldn't have done this work without the support and guidance of my association librarians and publisher.

I am especially grateful to Jo Milios, who collaborated with me on this project and is a devoted practitioner of prostate cancer physiotherapy and a strong advocate for men's health physiotherapy worldwide. I also want to thank my family, particularly my husband, for being my rock throughout this process and for his unwavering support and understanding, especially when I needed to prioritize writing over other responsibilities.

Lastly, I want to acknowledge my grandfather, Orlando Baiocchi, who passed away from prostate cancer in 1997. He was a medical professional who prioritized his patients' wellness above his own, often attending to them in a wheelchair due to his bone metastasis. His selflessness and unwavering commitment to his patients have been a constant source of motivation for me.

Writing this book has been an incredible journey, and I am grateful to everyone who has supported me along the way. I hope that this book serves as a source of inspiration and knowledge for many physiotherapists and oncology professionals, and that it will make a positive impact in the lives of individuals and families affected by prostate cancer.

GENDER LANGUAGE DISCLAIMER

This book uses the word "male" or "man" as a context of individuals whose sex assigned at birth was male, whether they identify as female, male, or non-binary.

Preface

Prostate cancer (PC) is the second most common form of cancer in men worldwide, and in 2020 about 1.4 million new cases of prostate cancer were reported.[1]

The survival rate for men diagnosed with prostate cancer is very high in developed countries, such as Australia, New Zealand, Northern and Western Europe (e.g., Norway, Sweden, Ireland), and North America (particularly in the United States).[2] In the UK, the estimated 10-year survival rate is about 78%, and in the United States and Canada the five-year estimated survival rate was about 93–96% in 2020.[3, 4, 5] The number of prostate cancer survivors (men who are still receiving or who have received cancer treatments) is growing worldwide, partly due to an increasing aging population (over 60% of PC survivors are over 70 years old) and early detection and treatment. In the United States alone, an estimated three million men live with prostate cancer.[6]

Unfortunately, prostate cancer treatments—including radical prostatectomy, radiation, and hormonal therapy (androgen deprivation therapy)—have side-effects which can immensely impact men's emotional state and overall quality of life. These are side-effects which, in most circumstances, can be addressed, minimized, or treated. Also, the knowledge of the disease and the expected future risks can cause mental distress and a reduction in the quality of life of men living with prostate cancer.[7] Shifting the focus to consider *all aspects* of cancer diagnosis and treatment and how they affect cancer survivors can help physiotherapists and oncology clinicians to properly identify risks, treatment efficacy to improve health-related quality of life, in addition to "quantity" of life.

Mental health concerns should take special consideration when addressing this population as psychological distress has been highly reported, for example, one in six men who is diagnosed with PC is likely to suffer from

---

1   (Sung *et al.*, 2021)
2   (Bray *et al.*, 2018)
3   (Cancer Research UK: Prostate Cancer Statistics, n.d.)
4   (Prostate Cancer in Canada, 2021)
5   (National Cancer Institute, n.d.)
6   (DeSantis *et al.*, 2014)
7   (Sennfält *et al.*, 2004)

clinically significant depression.[8] Psychosocial support and interventions have also been shown to improve prostate cancer patients' mental and physical health and quality of life and may even delay tumor progression and metastasis .[9, 10, 11] Additionally, oncology workers' psychological wellness may strengthen their own psychological resilience, promote compassion care, increase job satisfaction, and improve patients' outcomes.[12, 13]

By creating a greater understanding of the complexities of prostate cancer and the significant impact it can have on patients and their loved ones, healthcare professionals such as physiotherapists and cancer clinicians may be better-positioned to provide support and guidance to this population. Additionally, taking a comprehensive approach to prostate cancer survivorship, which includes addressing physical, emotional, and social needs, can greatly enhance the chances of individuals maintaining a high quality of life and achieving their goals beyond cancer treatment. In other words, caring for this population using a biopsychosocial humanist model can address all health domains that influence prostate cancer survivors' overall health, wellbeing, and mortality.

This book has been developed to help oncology professionals, cancer survivors, and their families to broaden their view on prostate cancer care based on evidence, research, and clinical experience. The goal of this book is to provide valuable insights and information that can help improve the management of side-effects resulting from prostate cancer treatments, with a focus on a more holistic biopsychosocial approach to care that considers the whole person and their unique needs. This book will cover a wide range of topics relevant to prostate cancer treatment and survivorship, including the latest research on treatment options and potential side-effects, as well as the importance of psychosocial interventions, exercise therapy, social support, and the physiology of the male pelvis, including the anatomy and function of pelvic floor muscles. Additionally, the book will explore the physiological changes that occur after treatment, offer novel approaches to pre- and post-prostatectomy rehabilitation, and provide conservative treatment strategies for bladder, bowel, and sexual health.

This book's intention is to suggest a different outlook on prostate cancer survivorship care, by introducing strategies to develop a compassionate, client-focused, culturally sensitive, humanistic biopsychosocial model of care.

8   (Fervaha *et al.*, 2019)
9   (Jacobsen & Jim, 2008)
10 (Chien *et al.*, 2014)
11 (Costanzo *et al.*, 2011)
12 (Neff *et al.*, 2020)
13 (Di Mario *et al.*, 2023)

REFERENCES

Bray, F., Ferlay, J., Soerjomataram, I., Siegel, R.L., Torre, L.A., & Jemal, A. (2018). Global cancer statistics 2018: GLOBOCAN estimates of incidence and mortality worldwide for 36 cancers in 185 countries. *CA: A Cancer Journal for Clinicians, 68*(6), 394-424. https://doi.org/10.3322/caac.21492

Cancer Research UK (n.d.). Prostate Cancer Statistics. https://www.cancerresearchuk.org/health-professional/cancer-statistics/statistics-by-cancer-type/prostate-cancer

Chien, C.-H., Liu, K.-L., Chien, H.-T., & Liu, H.-E. (2014). The effects of psychosocial strategies on anxiety and depression of patients diagnosed with prostate cancer: A systematic review. *International Journal of Nursing Studies, 51*(1), 28-38. https://doi.org/10.1016/j.ijnurstu.2012.12.019

Costanzo, E.S., Sood, A.K., & Lutgendorf, S.K. (2011). Biobehavioral influences on cancer progression. *Immunology and Allergy Clinics, 31*(1), 109-132. https://doi.org/10.1016/j.iac.2010.09.001

DeSantis, C.E., Lin, C.C., Mariotto, A.B., Siegel, R.L., et al. (2014). Cancer treatment and survivorship statistics, 2014. *CA: A Cancer Journal for Clinicians, 64*(4), 252-271. https://doi.org/10.3322/caac.21235

Di Mario, S., Cocchiara, R.A., & La Torre, G. (2023). The use of yoga and mindfulness-based interventions to reduce stress and burnout in healthcare workers: An umbrella review. *Alternative Therapies in Health and Medicine, 29*(1), 29-35.

Fervaha, G., Izard, J.P., Tripp, D.A., Rajan, S., Leong, D.P., & Siemens, D.R. (2019). Depression and prostate cancer: A focused review for the clinician. *Urologic Oncology, 37*(4), 282-288. https://doi.org/10.1016/j.urolonc.2018.12.020

Jacobsen, P.B., & Jim, H.S. (2008). Psychosocial interventions for anxiety and depression in adult cancer patients: Achievements and challenges. *CA: A Cancer Journal for Clinicians, 58*(4), 214-230. https://doi.org/10.3322/CA.2008.0003

National Cancer Institute (n.d.). Cancer Stat Facts: Prostate Cancer. https://seer.cancer.gov/statfacts/html/prost.html.

Neff, K.D., Knox, M.C., Long, P., & Gregory, K. (2020). Caring for others without losing yourself: An adaptation of the Mindful Self-Compassion Program for Healthcare Communities. *Journal of Clinical Psychology, 76*(9), 1543-1562. https://doi.org/10.1002/jclp.23007

Prostate Cancer in Canada (2021, March 17). https://www.canada.ca/en/public-health/services/publications/diseases-conditions/prostate-cancer.html

Sennfält, K., Carlsson, P., Sandblom, G., & Varenhorst, E. (2004). The estimated economic value of the welfare loss due to prostate cancer pain in a defined population. *Acta Oncologica (Stockholm, Sweden), 43*(3), 290-296. https://doi.org/10.1080/02841860410028411

Sung, H., Ferlay, J., Siegel, R.L., Laversanne, M., Soerjomataram, I., Jemal, A., & Bray, F. (2021). Global Cancer Statistics 2020: GLOBOCAN estimates of incidence and mortality worldwide for 36 cancers in 185 countries. *CA: A Cancer Journal for Clinicians, 71*(3), 209-249. https://doi.org/10.3322/caac.21660

PART 1

UNDERSTANDING PROSTATE CANCER TREATMENTS AND EFFECTS

CHAPTER 1

Prostate Cancer Treatments

Prostate cancer (PC) is the most common type of male cancer being diagnosed worldwide,[1] and it is the number one type of malignancy being diagnosed in over 50% of countries in the world.[2, 3] Fortunately, in the majority of cases, prostate cancer tends to grow slowly and be treated while still in a localized form, increasing the chances of survival. In the US and Canada, PC's five-year survival rate ranges from 93% to 96%.[4, 5, 6] PC treatments include active surveillance, surgery or removal of the prostate, radiation therapy, chemotherapy, and androgen deprivation therapy, and are dependent on many factors, such as: stage at diagnosis, risk of recurrence, patient's age, presence of comorbidities, and patient's personal preference.[7]

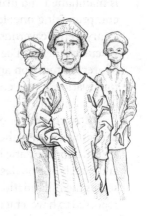

By providing a comprehensive overview of the various prostate cancer treatments and their potential impacts, this chapter aims to equip physiotherapists and oncology clinicians with the knowledge and resources needed to deliver optimal care and support to prostate cancer survivors throughout their recovery journey.

PROSTATECTOMY SURGERY

Radical prostatectomy (RP) surgery (removal of the entire prostate) is performed to treat localized or regional prostate cancer, and has the best incidence of survival rate of all prostate cancer treatments.[8] There are different types of radical prostatectomy procedures: laparoscopic, robotic,

1   (Mattiuzzi & Lippi, 2019)
2   (Sung et al., 2021)
3   (Leslie et al., 2022)
4   (Cancer Research UK, n.d.)
5   (Prostate Cancer in Canada, 2021)
6   (National Cancer Institute, n.d.)
7   (Miller et al., 2019)
8   (Serrell et al., 2018)

retropubic, and nerve sparing. Usually, the type of procedure is dependent on the surgeon's expertise and/or preference. There seems to be no difference in post-surgical outcome after six weeks of surgery between robotic, laparoscopic, and retropubic.[9]

During a radical prostatectomy the surgeon's main objective is to remove the cancer with clear surgical margins. Occasionally, nerve bundles and adjacent glands are also removed to lessen the chances of the cancer spreading. Once the prostate is removed, the bladder and the urethra are reattached (anastomosis) and a catheter is put in place for about 7–10 days, so the orifice is maintained and urination can occur after removal of the catheter. If not compromising oncologic efficacy, surgeons will try to spare or minimize injury to the cavernosal nerves and prostatic neurovascular supply (neurovascular bundle). The neurovascular bundle is important for preservation of erectile function and urinary continence, as they supply blood flow and innervation to the corpora cavernosa in the penis, rectum, prostate, and levator ani muscles.[10]

Most recently, novel approaches which may aid in recovery are being performed, such as the "hood" technique, where preservation of the detrusor apron, puboprostatic ligament complex, arcus tendineus, endopelvic fascia, and pouch of Douglas is achieved.[11, 12] Also the FFLU technique, which preserves the full functional length of the external urethral sphincter, has been reported to have a higher prevalence of urinary continence at one week post catheter removal compared to control.[13]

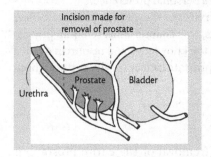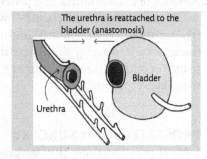

FIGURE 1.1: ILLUSTRATION OF A PROSTATECTOMY SURGERY

---

9   (Muaddi *et al.*, 2021)
10   (Costello *et al.*, 2004)
11   (Wagaskar *et al.*, 2021)
12   (Park *et al.*, 2013)
13   (Schlomm *et al.*, 2011)

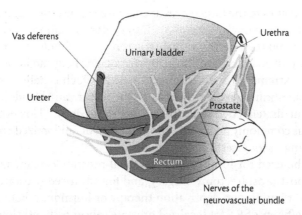

Vas deferens

Urethra

Urinary bladder

Ureter

Prostate

Rectum

Nerves of the
neurovascular bundle

FIGURE 1.2: THE NEUROVASCULAR BUNDLE (NVB)

RADIATION THERAPY

Radiation therapy (RT) or radiotherapy uses high energy rays to destroy cancer DNA cells. This can be applied extracorporeally (external beam radiation) or intracorporeally (such as brachytherapy). Brachytherapy is the implantation of radioactive seeds, which are placed interstitially to the prostate. Low-dose rate brachytherapy (LDRB) is usually performed for those diagnosed with low-to moderate-risk prostate cancer. This technique is used when the seeds are implanted in a course of several months, delivering radiation at a low dose per unit time.[14] Highly radioactive isotopes of iridium placed transperineally for a few minutes (high-dose rate brachytherapy) can also be used in combination with external beam radiation to treat high-risk prostate cancer.[15] The 17-year survival rate of those treated with LDRB for low to moderate risk PC was reported to be 97%,[16] and about one-third of US prostate cancer patients submitted to radiotherapy choose this form of treatment.[17]

External beam radiation delivers radiation in the form of x-rays, protons, or electrons three-dimensionally in order to limit exposure to tissues other than the prostate. To help limit healthy tissue exposure, external beam radiation most commonly is applied in large cumulative doses, via small daily fractions delivered over several weeks.[18] Technological advancements, such as Three-Dimensional Conformal Radiation Therapy (3-DCRT) and Intensity Modulated Radiation Therapy (IMRT), allow improvement in target coverage while reducing the dosage to healthy organs.[19] IMRT can be programmed to

---

14   (Bratt, 2007)
15   (Bratt, 2007)
16   (Lazarev *et al.*, 2018)
17   (Bratt, 2007)
18   (Martin & D'Amico, 2014)
19   (Martin & D'Amico, 2014)

vary the intensities to the targeted areas compared to healthy organs, as well as conform better to one's anatomy, with steep dose variations between the targeted area and the nearby normal structures.[20] Technological improvements in the past 20 years have also made stereotactic body radiation therapy (SBRT)—an extreme form of hypofractionation which is delivered in 4–7 fractions—significantly reduce the dose to the rectum and bladder, making the treatment also effective and with low rates of toxicity.[21] However, SBRT may not be as commonly prescribed due to the lack of randomized controlled trials assessing its long-term effectiveness.[22]

RT can be used for localized and regional prostate cancer, as salvage treatment post prostatectomy surgery, and for advanced prostate cancer combined with androgen deprivation therapy or hormonal therapy. Even though the efficacy of RT for localized prostate cancer is slightly lower than radical prostatectomy,[23] this choice of treatment is usually made in order to avoid side-effects from prostatectomy surgery.

ANDROGEN DEPRIVATION THERAPY

Androgen deprivation therapy (ADT) is mostly indicated to use in conjunction with radiation therapy in high-risk prostate cancer patients or to help shrink or delay cancer growth in metastatic prostate cancer.[24] The goal of ADT is to reduce the levels of androgens (male hormones) which are responsible for the growth of prostate cells, including cancer cells. Although ADT is not a form of curative treatment, it has been shown to improve quality of life and to reduce morbidity in metastatic prostate cancer.[25]

CHEMOTHERAPY

Chemotherapy drugs can be used to treat metastatic prostate cancer. Taxanes are often used as a front-line therapy for metastatic cancers such as breast, lung, ovarian, and prostate cancer. They can also be used in combination with other chemotherapy drugs or with radiation therapy to increase their effectiveness. Docetaxel and paclitaxel are two of the most commonly used taxanes. These drugs work by disrupting the normal function of microtubules, which are structures that help cells divide and replicate. By interfering with microtubules, taxanes prevent cancer cells from dividing and growing, leading to their death. In addition to its low systemic toxicity and

---

20 (Cho, 2018)
21 (Jackson *et al.*, 2019)
22 (Jacobs *et al.*, 2020)
23 (Serrell *et al.*, 2018)
24 (Pagliarulo *et al.*, 2012)
25 (Pagliarulo *et al.*, 2012)

higher cellular retention, docetaxel has been shown to improve overall survival rates and quality of life for patients with metastatic castration-resistant prostate cancer.[26]

Not all prostate cancer patients will be good candidates for chemotherapy treatments due to the possibility of chemoresistance and a range of potential side-effects, such as: decreased white blood cells production, increased risk for infection, nausea, vomiting, hair loss, mouth sores, easy bruising or bleeding, diarrhoea,[27] and increased risk of developing chemotherapy induced peripheral neuropathy (CIPN).[28] More on CIPN will be discussed in Chapter 4.

CANCER RISK ASSESSMENT: PROSTATE SPECIFIC ANTIGEN (PSA)

Blood markers, tumor classification, and pattern of prostate cells can be used to determine treatment approaches. PSA or prostate specific antigen is a blood test, which, with the combination of pathology reports, can be used as prostate cancer screening. The PSA number can be correlated to PSA surgical margin status and pathological state, and can be a predictor of recurring PSA post-surgery.[29] PSA testing is usually used post-surgically as a predictor of treatment success and treatment follow-up. After removal of the prostate, PSA levels in the blood should be undetectable after 6–8 weeks of surgery; if PSA levels are detectable (exceeding 0.1–0.2 ng/mL) and start to rise, then further treatment is recommended.[30]

GLEASON CLASSIFICATION SYSTEM

The Gleason score is used for adenocarcinoma[31] (most common form of prostate cancer) classification. It looks at cancer cell differentiation and arrangement, and it gives a score of 1–5, where the higher the score the more likely the cancer is to grow and spread. The score is calculated by adding the most common pattern score with the highest-grade pattern score.

---

26 (Konoshenko & Laktionov, 2022)
27 (Konoshenko & Laktionov, 2022)
28 (Ewertz *et al.*, 2015)
29 (Jones *et al.*, 2006)
30 (Cornford *et al.*, 2021)
31 (Murtagh *et al.*, 2018)

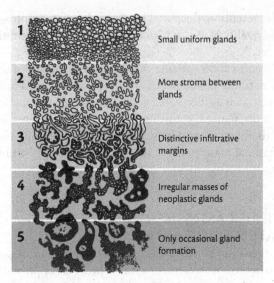

FIGURE I.3: GLEASON SCORE PATTERN[32]

Table I.I: Digital rectal examination (DRE) tumor node metastasis (TNM) classification[33]

To	No evidence of prostate tumor
T1	Not palpable, non-apparent tumor
T1a	Tumor incidental histological finding in 5% or less of tissue resected
T1b	Tumor incidental histological finding in more than 5% of tissue resected
T1c	Tumor identified by needle biopsy (i.e., due to elevated PSA)
T2	Tumor that is palpable and confined within the prostate
T2a	Tumor involves one half of one lobe or less
T2b	Tumor involves more than half of one lobe, but not both lobes
T2c	Tumor involves both lobes
T3	Tumor extends through the prostatic capsule
T3a	Extracapsular extension (unilateral or bilateral)
T3b	Tumor invades seminal vesicle(s)
T4	Tumor is fixed or invades other adjacent structures (e.g., external sphincter, rectum, levator ani muscles)

---

32 (Epstein, 2010)
33 (Cornford *et al.*, 2021)

Table 1.2: European Association of Urology (EAU) and the European Association of Nuclear Medicine (EANM) prostate cancer risk groups[34]

Low Risk	Intermediate Risk	High Risk	
PSA <10 ng/mL and GS <7 and T1–2a	PSA >10–20 ng/mL or GS=7 or T2b	PSA >20 ng/mL or GS >7 or T2c	Any PSA Any GS T3–T4
Localized			Advanced

PSA = prostate-specific antigen   GS = Gleason score

REFERENCES

Bratt, O. (2007). The urologist's guide to low dose-rate interstitial brachytherapy with permanent seed implants for localized prostate cancer. *BJU International, 99*(3), 497–501. https://doi.org/10.1111/j.1464-410X.2006.06587.x

Cancer Research UK (n.d.). Prostate cancer statistics. https://www.cancerresearchuk.org/health-professional/cancer-statistics/statistics-by-cancer-type/prostate-cancer#:~:text=There%20are%20around%2052%2C300%20new,UK%20(2016%2D2018)

Cancer Stat Facts (n.d.). Prostate Cancer [National Cancer Institute: Surveillance, Epidimiology and End Results program]. https://seer.cancer.gov/statfacts/html/prost.html

Cho, B. (2018). Intensity-modulated radiation therapy: A review with a physics perspective. *Radiation Oncology Journal, 36*(1), 1–10. https://doi.org/10.3857/roj.2018.00122

Cornford, P., van den Bergh, R.C.N., Briers, E., Van den Broeck, T., et al. (2021). EAU-EANM-ESTRO-ESUR-SIOG Guidelines on Prostate Cancer. Part II—2020 Update: Treatment of Relapsing and Metastatic Prostate Cancer. *European Urology, 79*(2), 263–282. https://doi.org/10.1016/j.eururo.2020.09.046

Costello, A.J., Brooks, M., & Cole, O.J. (2004). Anatomical studies of the neurovascular bundle and cavernosal nerves. *BJU International, 94*(7), 961–1182. Retrieved July 6, 2022, from https://bjui-journals.onlinelibrary.wiley.com/doi/10.1111/j.1464-410X.2004.05106.x

Epstein, J.I. (2010). An update of the Gleason grading system. *Journal of Urology, 183*(2), 433–440. https://doi.org/10.1016/j.juro.2009.10.046

Ewertz, M., Qvortrup, C., & Eckhoff, L. (2015). Chemotherapy-induced peripheral neuropathy in patients treated with taxanes and platinum derivatives. *Acta Oncologica, 54*(5), 587–591. https://doi.org/10.3109/0284186X.2014.995775

Jackson, W.C., Silva, J., Hartman, H.E., Dess, R.T., et al. (2019). Stereotactic body radiation therapy for localized prostate cancer: A systematic review and meta-analysis of over 6,000 patients treated on prospective studies. *International Journal of Radiation Oncology, Biology, Physics, 104*(4), 778–789. https://doi.org/10.1016/j.ijrobp.2019.03.051

Jacobs, B.L., Hamm, M., de Abril Cameron, F., Luiggi-Hernandez, J.G., Heron, D.E., Kahn, J.M., & Barnato, A.E. (2020). Radiation oncologists' attitudes and beliefs about intensity-modulated radiation therapy and stereotactic body radiation therapy for prostate cancer. *BMC Health Services Research, 20*(1), 796. https://doi.org/10.1186/s12913-020-05656-x

Jones, T.D., Koch, M.O., Bunde, P.J., & Cheng, L. (2006). Is prostate-specific antigen (PSA) density better than the preoperative PSA level in predicting early biochemical recurrence of prostate cancer after radical prostatectomy? *BJU International, 97*(3), 480–484. https://doi.org/10.1111/j.1464-410X.2006.06022.x

Konoshenko, M., & Laktionov, P. (2022). The miRNAs involved in prostate cancer chemotherapy response as chemoresistance and chemosensitivity predictors. *Andrology, 10*(1), 51–71. https://doi.org/10.1111/andr.13086

---

34 (Cornford *et al.*, 2021)

Lazarev, S., Thompson, M.R., Stone, N.N., & Stock, R.G. (2018). Low-dose-rate brachytherapy for prostate cancer: Outcomes at >10 years of follow-up. *BJU International, 121*(5), 781–790. https://doi.org/10.1111/bju.14122

Leslie, S.W., Soon-Sutton, T.L., Sajjad, H., & Siref, L.E. (2022). Prostate cancer. In *StatPearls*. StatPearls Publishing. http://www.ncbi.nlm.nih.gov/books/NBK470550/

Martin, N.E., & D'Amico, A.V. (2014). Progress and controversies: Radiation therapy for prostate cancer. *CA: A Cancer Journal for Clinicians, 64*(6), 389–407. https://doi.org/10.3322/caac.21250

Mattiuzzi, C., & Lippi, G. (2019). Current cancer epidemiology. *Journal of Epidemiology and Global Health, 9*(4), 217–222. https://doi.org/10.2991/jegh.k.191008.001

Miller, K.D., Nogueira, L., Mariotto, A.B., Rowland, J.H., *et al.* (2019). Cancer treatment and survivorship statistics, 2019. *CA: A Cancer Journal for Clinicians, 69*(5), 363–385. https://doi.org/10.3322/caac.21565

Muaddi, H., Hafid, M.E., Choi, W.J., Lillie, E., *et al.* (2021). Clinical outcomes of robotic surgery compared to conventional surgical approaches (laparoscopic or open): A systematic overview of reviews. *Annals of Surgery, 273*(3), 467–473. https://doi.org/10.1097/SLA.0000000000003915

Murtagh, J., Rosenblatt, J., Murtagh, C., & Coleman, J. (2018). *Murtagh's General Practice, 7th edition.* Sydney, NSW: McGraw-Hill Education.

Pagliarulo, V., Bracarda, S., Eisenberger, M.A., Mottet, N., Schröder, F.H., Sternberg, C., & Studer, U.E. (2012). Contemporary role of androgen deprivation therapy for prostate cancer. *European Urology, 61*(1), 11–25. https://doi.org/10.1016/j.eururo.2011.08.026

Park, Y.H., Jeong, C.W., & Lee, S.E. (2013). A comprehensive review of neuroanatomy of the prostate. *Prostate International, 1*(4), 139–145. https://doi.org/10.12954/PI.13020

Prostate Cancer in Canada. (2021, March 17). https://www.canada.ca/en/public-health/services/publications/diseases-conditions/prostate-cancer.html

Schlomm, T., Heinzer, H., Steuber, T., Salomon, G., *et al.* (2011). Full functional-length urethral sphincter preservation during radical prostatectomy. *European Urology, 60*(2), 320–329. https://doi.org/10.1016/j.eururo.2011.02.040

Serrell, E.C., Pitts, D., Hayn, M., Beaule, L., Hansen, M.H., & Sammon, J.D. (2018). Review of the comparative effectiveness of radical prostatectomy, radiation therapy, or expectant management of localized prostate cancer in registry data. *Urologic Oncology, 36*(4), 183–192. https://doi.org/10.1016/j.urolonc.2017.10.003

Sung, H., Ferlay, J., Siegel, R.L., Laversanne, M., Soerjomataram, I., Jemal, A., & Bray, F. (2021). Global Cancer Statistics 2020: GLOBOCAN Estimates of Incidence and Mortality Worldwide for 36 Cancers in 185 Countries. *CA: A Cancer Journal for Clinicians, 71*(3), 209–249. https://doi.org/10.3322/caac.21660

Wagaskar, V.G., Mittal, A., Sobotka, S., Ratnani, P., *et al.* (2021). Hood technique for robotic radical prostatectomy—Preserving periurethral anatomical structures in the space of retzius and sparing the Pouch of Douglas, enabling early return of continence without compromising surgical margin rates. *European Urology, 80*(2), 213–221. https://doi.org/10.1016/j.eururo.2020.09.044

The Anatomy and Physiology of the Male Pelvis

This chapter provides an overview of the male pelvis's anatomy and physiology, with a particular focus on information relevant to treating prostate cancer survivors with regard to bladder, bowel, and sexual function. Modernized technology has led to an increasing number of studies that review and update information on male pelvic anatomy. Traditional pelvic illustrations in textbooks are often based on cadaver studies, which can be distorted after the embalming process. As a result, these illustrations may not accurately depict what the pelvic floor muscles and related structures look like in clinical practice. Recently, 3D reconstruction models from magnetic resonance imaging and real-time ultrasound studies have provided greater accuracy in understanding the anatomical structures and function of the male pelvis, as well as providing more insights into male continence control and sexual function.

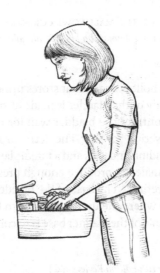

THE MALE LOWER URINARY TRACT

The male lower urinary tract consists of the urinary bladder, prostate, and urethra; its function is to store and voluntarily expel urine.

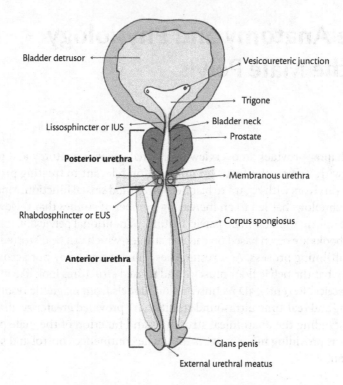

Bladder detrusor
Vesicoureteric junction
Trigone
Lissosphincter or IUS
Bladder neck
Prostate
Posterior urethra
Membranous urethra
Rhabdosphincter or EUS
Corpus spongiosus
Anterior urethra
Glans penis
External urethral meatus

FIGURE 2.1: THE MALE LOWER URINARY TRACT
Image owned by Samantha Hughes, all rights reserved

The urinary bladder

The urinary bladder is a hollow organ that stores urine and is composed of a body and a base. The body of the bladder is made of smooth muscles (detrusors) whose role is to contract the bladder wall for the expulsion of urine (parasympathetic innervation S2–S4).[1] The detrusor muscles have an inner and outer layer of longitudinal muscles and a middle layer of circular muscles,[2] and they are thicker in males to produce enough pressure in order to expel urine from the longer urethra.[3] The base of the bladder includes the trigone, a triangular shaped area where the ureter enters into the bladder and where the urethra begins. The role of the bladder base is to control urine flow, having

---

1   (*Campbell–Walsh Urology 11th Edition Review*, n.d.)
2   (Andersson & Arner, 2004)
3   (Abelson *et al.*, 2018)

parasympathetic and sympathetic stimulation to allow or prevent urination. The bladder neck (the area where the bladder meets the urethra) also shares a common border with the prostatic urethra[4], and it has higher concentration of adrenergic receptors that promote constriction of the bladder neck during ejaculation to prevent semen from entering the bladder.[5]

The bladder is retained in place by 5 true ligaments and 3–5 false ligaments (formed by peritoneal folds). It is a relatively free-floating organ, which is covered by the peritoneum superiorly and posteriorly, and by endopelvic fascia inferiorly and inferolaterally.[6, 7] In males the bladder neck is fixed in position by the puboprostatic ligament, which is an important ligament to preserve during prostatectomy surgery.[8]

The prostate

The prostate gland is a walnut-shaped organ flattened from front to back and can be divided into three layers from superior to inferior (base, midgland, and apex).[9] The *base* of the prostate is where the prostate connects with the urinary bladder at the bladder neck. It is also where the prostatic urethra begins and where the ejaculatory ducts enter the prostate. The *midgland* is the middle third of the prostate gland and the apex is where the prostatic urethra ends superiorly to the external urethral sphincter. The prostatic capsule fuses at the base with the bladder detrusor and at the apex with the external urethral sphincter.[10] However this capsule, which is made of condensed fibromuscular tissue, has different arrangements of fibrous and muscle tissue throughout the prostate, making it difficult to define the prostate borders (especially anteriorly).[11] The prostate is supported by a three-layered fascia system: the Denonvilliers' fascia, the prostatic fascia, and the endopelvic fascia. The Denonvilliers' fascia is found posteriorly to the prostate between the prostate and the rectum. The prostatic fascia surrounds the prostate posterior-laterally and it fuses laterally with the endopelvic fascia (figure 2.2).[12] The puboprostatic ligaments hold and attach the prostate to the pubic bone.[13] The blood and nerve supply to the prostate gland is housed in between the layers of the prostatic and endopelvic fascia.[14] The prostate gland's main function is to produce seminal fluid which protects and nourishes the semen.

4   (Mangera *et al.*, 2013)
5   (*Campbell-Walsh Urology 11th Edition Review,* n.d.)
6   (Gray, 1988)
7   (Mangera *et al.*, 2013)
8   (Ratanapornsompong *et al.*, 2021)
9   (Sklinda *et al.*, 2019)
10 (Sklinda *et al.*, 2019)
11 (Fine & Reuter, 2012)
12 (Raychaudhuri & Cahill, 2008)
13 (Choi *et al.*, 2020)
14 (Raychaudhuri & Cahill, 2008)

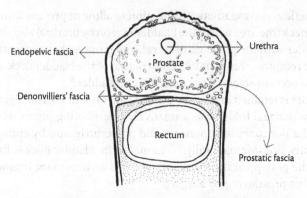

Endopelvic fascia

Prostate

Urethra

Denonvilliers' fascia

Rectum

Prostatic fascia

FIGURE 2.2: THE PROSTATIC FASCIA SYSTEM
*Adapted from Raychaudhuri & Cahill, 2008.[15] Image owned
by Samantha Hughes, all rights reserved*

The male urethra

The male urethra's role is to allow passage of urine and semen. It connects the urinary bladder to the outer orifice and it is divided into the posterior urethra (arising from the bladder neck to the urethral membrane) and the anterior urethra (from the urethral membrane distal to the prostate to the urethral meatus). Anteriorly the male urethra is supported by the pubovesical and puboprostatic ligament and the tendinous arch of the pelvic fascia, and posteriorly it is supported by the Denonvillier's fascia, the perineal body, and the levator ani complex (see pelvic floor section below).[16]

The male urethra also houses the urethral sphincter complex, the inner lissosphincter (internal urethral sphincter or IUS), and the outer rhabdo-sphincter (external urethral sphincter or EUS).[17] The main function of the urethral sphincters is to control urine storage.

According to Koraitim, the internal urethral sphincter (IUS) is made of circular smooth muscles surrounding the entire urethra, being most prominent at the opening of the bladder into the urethra (vesical orifice). The main role of the IUS is to maintain *passive continence*, mostly controlled at the bladder neck. The external urethral sphincter (EUS) is predominantly located distal to the prostate apex, with proximal fibers at the anterolateral side of the prostate. It is composed of striated muscle fibers containing a combination of slow and fast twitch muscle fibers. The distal part of the EUS is mostly responsible for active continence as when contracted it approximates the anterior urethral wall towards the posterior wall, consequently occluding the urethra. The proximal part of the EUS seems to be related to

---

15 (Raychaudhuri & Cahill, 2008)
16 (Rehder *et al.*, 2016)
17 (Koraitim, 2008)

sexual function by providing antegrated propulsion of semen, preventing retrograted ejaculation.[18]

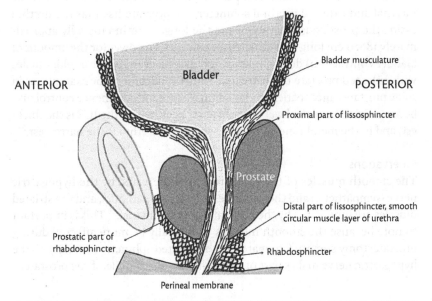

FIGURE 2.3: THE REVISED CONCEPT OF THE MALE URETHRAL SPHINCTER COMPLEX
*Modified and adapted from Koraitim, 2008.[19] Image owned
by Samantha Hughes, all rights reserved*

Micturition in males

The micturition process is complex and involves the integration of the autonomic, somatic, and central nervous system. In simple terms, urine is produced in the kidneys and transported to the urinary bladder to be stored. As described above, storage is possible due to the internal and external urethral sphincters. Normally, when the bladder is half-full, information is automatically sent from the bladder to nerves in the sacrum and back, contracting the bladder detrusor and relaxing the internal urethral sphincter (sacral parasympathetic innervation). This process is called the micturition reflex. To avoid involuntary urination, or as a response of increased intra-abdominal pressure, the external urethral sphincter contracts[20] (pudendal nerve innervation)—controlled by higher centers in the brain—inhibiting parasympathetic stimulation to the detrusor muscles, and making the bladder relax. When parasympathetic stimulation decreases, urine storage is possible

---

18 (Koraitim, 2008)
19 (Koraitim, 2008)
20 (Koraitim, 2008)

due to thoraco-lumbar sympathetic innervation that inhibits the bladder detrusor muscles while exciting the bladder base and urethra.[21]

There are many obstacles for urine passage in the male anatomy: the internal and external urethral sphincter, the prostate itself (as the urethra inside the prostate is narrower), and the longer urethra (usually approximately 18–20 cm long[22]). The detrusor contraction power (or the amount of bladder contraction) during micturition may be even higher in older males with enlarged prostate or obstructive outlet syndrome,[23] for example, as in some prostate cancer patients. Maximum closure and continence control may be assumed to be at the level of the bladder neck, where the IUS is the thickest, and in the membranous urethra, where the urethra is the narrowest.[24]

Innervations

The smooth muscles of the sphincters are innervated by the hypogastric nerve (sympathetic) and the pelvic nerve (parasympathetic), and the striated muscles are innervated by the pudendal nerve (somatic).[25] This is important to note because the smooth muscles will usually be more affected during prostatectomy surgery (compared to the striated sphincter muscles), as the hypogastric nerve makes part of the neurovascular bundle of the prostate.[26]

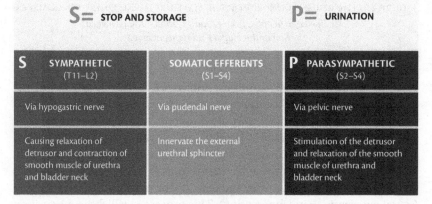

S= STOP AND STORAGE   P= URINATION

S SYMPATHETIC (T11–L2)	SOMATIC EFFERENTS (S1–S4)	P PARASYMPATHETIC (S2–S4)
Via hypogastric nerve	Via pudendal nerve	Via pelvic nerve
Causing relaxation of detrusor and contraction of smooth muscle of urethra and bladder neck	Innervate the external urethral sphincter	Stimulation of the detrusor and relaxation of the smooth muscle of urethra and bladder neck

FIGURE 2.4: BLADDER PHYSIOLOGY INNERVATIONS
Image owned by Samantha Hughes, all rights reserved

---

21   (de Groat, 2006)
22   (Abelson *et al.*, 2018)
23   (Rosier *et al.*, 1995)
24   (Koraitim, 2008)
25   (Creed, 1995)
26   (Hoeh *et al.*, 2022)

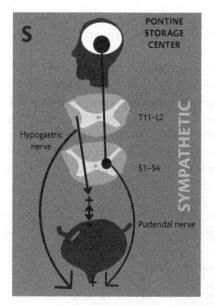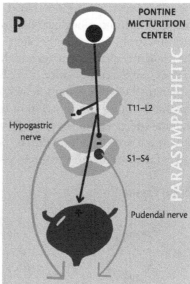

FIGURE 2.5: SYMPATHETIC AND PARASYMPATHETIC BLADDER CONTROL
Image owned by Samantha Hughes, all rights reserved

THE PENIS

The human penis is a unique structure to the male urinary and reproductive system. It consists of a *root,* a *body*, and the *glans penis* (extremity). The body of the penis is between the root and the glans penis and it contains the largest part of the urethra. The root is connected to the pubis and ischium by the crura (the proximal tapering of the corpora cavernosa) and the suspensory ligaments (which are an extension of the linea alba), and it is surrounded by the ischio-cavernosus muscles, beginning directly after the bulbourethral glands.[27, 28] The penis terminates at the glans penis, which is a widening of the corpus spongiosum, starting where the corpora cavernosa ends and where the urethra terminates (the urethral meatus) . When not erect or circumcized, the glans penis is sheathed by a circular skin-fold named the prepuce.[29]

Structurally, the penis is composed of three cylindrical "venous sinusoid" compartments surrounded by fascia—two corpora cavernosa superiorly (dorsal) and one corpus spongiosum inferiorly (ventral) which encloses the urethra.[30] These compartments are usually named erectile tissue, as the sinusoids are filled with blood during erections, the main erectile tissues being the duo corpora cavernosa. There is a partially fenestrating septum separating the

---

27 (Avery & Scheinfeld, 2013)
28 (Lindquist *et al.*, 2020)
29 (Gray, 1988)
30 (Gray, 1988)

two corpora cavernosa to allow blood to circulate between the two corpora cavernosa.[31] The tunica albuginea (TA) surrounding the two corpora cavernosa are thick and strong to sustain the high pressure being generated during erection. The triangular-shaped structures at the ventral thickening of the TA (from 5 to 7 o'clock) are the continuation of the bulbospongiosus muscles, and the dorsal thickening (between 11 and 1 o'clock) contains the ischiocavernosus muscles. Distally the outer continuation of the TA forms the distal ligament which supports the glans penis, especially when erect. The Buck's fascia separates the corpora cavernosa from the corpus spongiosum, and the most superficial Dartos fascia surrounds the three cylindrical compartments.[32]

Penile vessels[33]

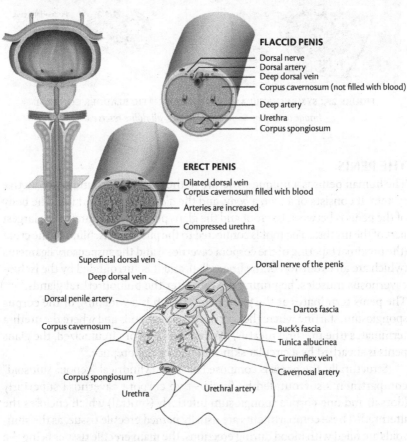

FIGURE 2.6: PENIS ANATOMY

Images from © 2003–2023 Shutterstock, Inc., standard licence

---

31 (Lindquist *et al.*, 2020)
32 (Lindquist *et al.*, 2020)
33 (Lindquist *et al.*, 2020)

Blood supply to the penis arises from the pudendal arteries (a branch of the hypogastric artery) supplying the perineal and common penile arteries—branched into bulbourethral artery, the dorsal artery of the penis, and the cavernosal artery. The bulbourethral artery supplies the bulbourethral gland, the urethral bulb, and the posterior aspect of the corpus spongiosum. The dorsal arteries supply the distal aspect of the corpus spongiosum and glans penis. The cavernosal artery courses through the center of the corpora cavernosa. The penile drainage mostly occurs via the superficial and deep dorsal veins, which are then drained into the internal pudendal vein.

The simplified physiology of penile erection[34, 35, 36]

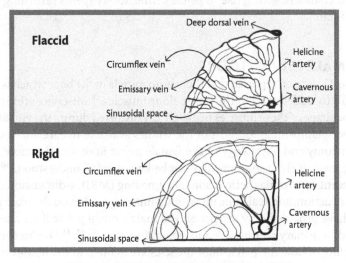

FIGURE 2.7: CORPUS CAVERNOSUM BLOOD VESSEL
REPRESENTATION DURING ERECT AND FLACCID STATE
*Adapted and modified from Anatomy and Physiology of Erection:
Pathophysiology of erectile dysfunction, 2003*[37]

Penile erection (*penile tumescence*) occurs through a neuro-hemodynamic process due to a variety of neurotransmitter stimulations, with autonomic and somatic innervations. Erection can occur from direct genital stimulation, nocturnally following rapid eye movement cycles, and centrally due to psychogenic stimulation. Parasympathetic stimulation (S1–S4) via the cavernous nerves induces relaxation of smooth muscles of the sinusoids, allowing increased blood flow to the sinusoids, stretching the tunica albuginea, and

---

34 ("Chapter 2," 2003, p. 2)
35 (Dean & Lue, 2005)
36 (Hsu, 2006)
37 ("Chapter 2," 2003, p.2)

compressing the veins in between the TA and the Buck's fascia, consequently reducing venous outflow (*full-erection phase*). Somatic stimulation contracts the ischiocavernosus muscles, further increasing the penile pressure, producing the *rigid-erection phase*. Venous compression happens mostly around the two corpora cavernosa as the TA is thicker and bi-layered and surrounds them entirely; penile pressure is not as high in the corpus spongiosum as the thinner TA and bulbospongiosus muscle only partially enclose it, allowing ejaculation to occur when the penis is erect. Ejaculation occurs with stimulation of the bulbospongiosus (deep branch of perineal nerve S2–S4). Sympathetic stimulation (T1–L2) causes smooth muscle contraction, which then produces a slow reduction of penile pressure with reopening of the venous channels, giving rise to *penile detumescence* (penis returning to its flaccid state).

THE MALE PELVIC FLOOR

In 1889, Dickinson reported that there is no muscle in the body which is more difficult to understand as the pelvic floor muscles.[38] Misconceptions arise due the shape of these muscles being greatly distorted during the embalming process.[39] Unfortunately, most of the studies available to date are based on the anatomy and physiology of the female pelvic floor and therefore, even today, "basic (pelvic) anatomy may not be known or all understood."[40]

Recent *in vivo* magnetic resonance imaging (MRI), 3-dimensional (3D) reconstruction, and real-time ultrasound imaging studies on the male pelvic floor have provided new insight on the male *striated* pelvic floor anatomy related to urinary continence and sexual function.[41, 42, 43] Due to the high variability of how the pelvic floor muscles are defined in the literature, this section will base the pelvic floor musculature definitions and terminology from the International Continence Society (ICS) "Report on the terminology for pelvic floor muscle assessment," published in 2021.[44]

The pelvic fascia

The pelvic floor musculature together with the obturator internus and piriformis muscles are enveloped by endopelvic fascia. The endopelvic fascia is a fascia layer covering the walls and floor of the pelvis and it is fused with the periosteum of the hipbone.[45] It can further be subdivided into the parietal and

38   (Dickinson, 1889)
39   (Shobeiri *et al.*, 2008)
40   (Patrick C. Walsh, quoted in Raychaudhuri & Cahill (2008))
41   (Bianchi *et al.*, 2018)
42   (Wu *et al.*, 2020)
43   (Tai *et al.*, 2021)
44   (Frawley *et al.*, 2021)
45   (Raychaudhuri & Cahill, 2008)

visceral layers; the first covering the wall of the pelvis and the last suspending the pelvic organs.[46] The endopelvic fascia merges laterally with the prostatic fascia,[47] and thickens in between the levator ani (LA) complex and the obturator internus forming the tendinous arch of the endopelvic fascia. The pelvic fascia is a three-dimensional structure composed of collagen, elastin, smooth muscles, blood vessels, nerves, and lymphatics.[48]

The levator ani complex

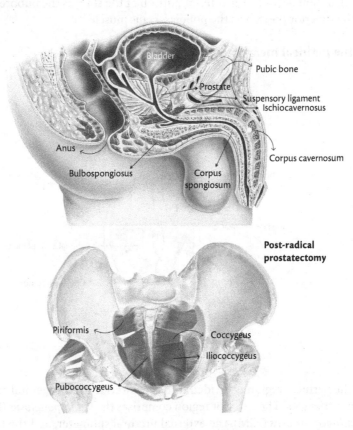

FIGURE 2.8: THE LEVATOR ANI MUSCLES
Images adapted from © 2003–2023 Shutterstock, Inc., standard licence

The levator ani complex includes the striated muscles: pubococcygeus, puborectalis, pubovisceralis, iliococcygeus, and ischiococcygeus/coccygeus (vestigial). The male LA complex originates from the pubis (body and superior

---

46   (Siccardi & Bordoni, 2022)
47   (Raychaudhuri & Cahill, 2008)
48   (Siccardi & Bordoni, 2022)

ramus) inserting on the tendinous arch of the levator ani muscle, the ramus of the ilium, ischium, the anus, the rectum, the deep perineal body, and the coccyx. It forms a horizontal sheet that helps support the pelvic viscera. This sheet seems to have a deeper funnel-shape and less pronounced "S"-shape of the distal rectum and anal canal compared to females, creating a more favorable leverage.[49] Some authors categorize the *puborectalis* as a "U"-shaped muscle originated at the pubic rami, running dorsally while creating a sling around the anus and the urethra.[50] Other authors were able to show a distinct separation between the inferior portion of the sling as the puborectalis and the superior portion as the pubovisceralis muscle.[51]

The perineal membrane and muscles

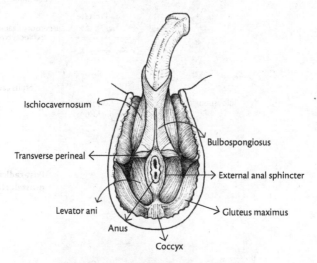

FIGURE 2.9: THE PERINEAL MUSCLES
Image owned by Samantha Hughes, all rights reserved.

The perineal region is divided into the anterior urethrogenital and posterior triangles. The anterior region comprises the *bulbospongiosus* (BSM), the *ischiocavernosus* (ICM), the external urethral sphincter, and the transverse perineal muscles (deep and superficial); and the posterior anal triangle comprises the *anal external sphincter*.[52] A mass of connective tissue with no distinctive border located between the bulb of the penis and the anus is called the *perineal body*. The superficial part of the perineal body serves as attachments to the superficial transverse perineal and the bulbospongiosus

49   (Wu *et al.*, 2020)
50   (Tai *et al.*, 2021)
51   (Wu *et al.*, 2020)
52   (Siccardi & Bordoni, 2022)

muscles.[53] The bulbospongiosus originates from the perineal body, the medial raphe, and the corpus cavernosum inserting into the tunica albuginea, corpus spongiosum and the *levator ani muscles*.[54] Its middle fibers also surround the bulb of the urethra and contribute to emptying urine from the urethra once the bladder has emptied.[55] Recent studies also suggested that a superficial area of the anal external sphincter and the BSM are connected and share the same innervation.[56, 57] The ischiocavernosus is paired and located at the lateral boundary of the perineum, originated at the ischial tuberosity, running along the medial and lateral border of each crus (tapering of the corpora cavernosa) attaching to the tunica albuginea.[58] At the penile crura, both ICM and the BSM encircle their corresponding body—the corpora cavernosa and corpus spongiosum respectively.

The anal sphincter muscles, mostly innervated by the pudendal nerve, are composed of elliptical muscular fibers surrounding the margins of the anus, arising from the coccyx and inserting into the perineal body. [59] These muscles share synergistic actions with the puborectalis muscles.[60]

The pelvic floor function: A review

The pelvic floor, composed of pelvic muscles, ligaments, and fascia, occludes the pelvic outlet, leaving orifices for the rectum and the urethra to pass the perineum.[61] The pelvic floor striated muscles receive somatic innervations from the sacral plexus (S2–S4) and the pudendal nerve.[62] They contain a constant resting tone, and contract in response to increased intra-abdominal pressure to increase urethral and anal sphincter closure function.[63] There are usually constant adjustments made by these muscles in response to change of activities. They are dynamic structures contracting and relaxing at appropriate times: contracting to increase closure to the anus and urethra together with elevating the pelvis in a cranial–ventral direction, and relaxing to allow urination and defecation to occur. [64] Ultrasound imaging studies were able to demonstrate a cranial displacement of the bladder base at the urethrovesical junction, a caudal displacement of the mid-urethra, and compression of the bulb of the penis during voluntary pelvic floor muscle

53   (Wu *et al.*, 2020)
54   (Hsu *et al.*, 2004)
55   (Siccardi & Bordoni, 2022)
56   (Suriyut *et al.*, 2020)
57   (Plochocki *et al.*, 2016)
58   (Hsu *et al.*, 2004)
59   (Gray, 1988)
60   (Andromanakos *et al.*, 2020)
61   (Andromanakos *et al.*, 2020)
62   (Bharucha, 2006)
63   (Tai *et al.*, 2021)
64   (Talasz *et al.*, 2022)

contraction.[65] In males these movements can be best explained by activation of the levator ani, the external urethral sphincter, and the bulbospongiosus muscles respectively, providing insight on how the continence mechanism is supported by these muscles.[66] The puborectalis portion of the levator ani when contracted pulls the anorectal junction in a ventral direction, and its tonic activity influences the ventral curvature in the rectum.[67] It has been noted that there is a decreased ventral movement of the rectum towards the pubis of those suffering from urinary incontinence post-prostatectomy, supporting the role of the puborectalis muscle in being part of the urinary continence system in males.[68]

Tai *et al.*'s study demonstrated the role of the ischiocavernosus muscles in helping to occlude penile veins during erection, and also theorized that weak ICM could lead to decreased constriction to the dorsal vein causing venous leakage and decreased erection.[69] ICM contraction maximizes corpora cavernosal rigidity by compressing the roots of the corpora cavernosa, while bulbospongiosus muscles maximize corpus spongiosum rigidity by engorgement of the bulb of the penis.[70] The BSM contracts at the end of micturition after the bladder is emptied and also contracts during ejaculation when the bulb of the penis is engorged.[71]

The external anal sphincter (EAS), together with the puborectalis muscle and the internal anal sphincter (IAS), compose the fecal continence musculature mechanism. The EAS controls about 20–30% of the anal resting tone as well as the voluntary continence mechanism, contracting reflexively and voluntarily once fecal matter enters the rectum.[72]

Table 2.1: The role of the pelvic floor complex

Role	Mechanism
Support pelvic organs	Shape, location, and attachments of the LA, pelvic fascia, and ligaments
Help to maximize erection	Compressing the roots of the corpora cavernosa by the ICM and engorging the bulb of the penis by the BSM[73]

65 (Stafford *et al.*, 2014)
66 (Stafford *et al.*, 2012)
67 (Stafford *et al.*, 2014)
68 (Kumagai *et al.*, 2022)
69 (Tai *et al.*, 2021)
70 (Cohen *et al.*, 2016)
71 (Tanahashi *et al.*, 2012)
72 (Patel *et al.*, 2021)
73 (Cohen *et al.*, 2016)

Support the continent urinary mechanism	Tonicity of the EUS[74] Contraction of LA, BSM, and EUS with increased intra-abdominal pressure[75, 76]
Clear urine in the urethra after bladder emptying	Contraction of BSM at the end of urination
Ejaculation	Expulsion of the semen occurs with relaxation of the bladder neck and EUS with multiple contraction bursts of BSM, ICM, LA, and perineal muscles[77, 78]
Prevent retrograde ejaculation	Contraction of the proximal part of the EUS [79]
Fecal continence mechanism	Resting tone of the EAS, IAS, and puborectalis and voluntary action of the EAS and puborectalis[80]

REFERENCES

Abelson, B., Sun, D., Que, L., Nebel, R.A., et al. (2018). Sex differences in lower urinary tract biology and physiology. Biology of Sex Differences, 9(1), 45. https://doi.org/10.1186/s13293-018-0204-8

Andersson, K.-E., & Arner, A. (2004). Urinary bladder contraction and relaxation: Physiology and pathophysiology. Physiological Reviews, 84(3), 935–986. https://doi.org/10.1152/physrev.00038.2003

Andromanakos, N., Filippou, D., Karandreas, N., & Kostakis, A. (2020). Puborectalis muscle and external anal sphincter: A functional unit? Turkish Journal of Gastroenterology, 31(4), 342–343. https://doi.org/10.5152/tjg.2020.19208

Avery, L.L., & Scheinfeld, M.H. (2013). Imaging of penile and scrotal emergencies. RadioGraphics, 33(3), 721–740. https://doi.org/10.1148/rg.333125158

Bharucha, A.E. (2006). Pelvic floor: Anatomy and function. Neurogastroenterology and Motility, 18(7), 507–519. https://doi.org/10.1111/j.1365-2982.2006.00803.x

Bianchi, L., Turri, F. M., Larcher, A., De Groote, R., et al. A. (2018). A novel approach for apical dissection during robot-assisted radical prostatectomy: The "collar" technique. European Urology Focus, 4(5), 677–685. https://doi.org/10.1016/j.euf.2018.01.004

Campbell–Walsh Urology 11th Edition Review—Elsevier eBook on VitalSource, 2nd Edition (9780323680714) (n.d.). Retrieved August 2, 2022, from https://evolve.elsevier.com/cs/product/9780323680714?role=student

Chapter 2: Anatomy and Physiology of erection: pathophysiology of erectile dysfunction. (2003). International Journal of Impotence Research, 15(7), S5–S8. https://doi.org/10.1038/sj.ijir.3901127

Choi, H.-M., Jung, S.-Y., Kim, S.-J., Yang, H.-J., et al. (2020). Clinical anatomy of the puboprostatic ligament for the safe guidance for the prostate surgery. Urology, 136, 190–195. https://doi.org/10.1016/j.urology.2019.10.015

---

74 (Yalla et al., 1979)
75 (Stafford et al., 2014)
76 (Koraitim, 2008)
77 (Tanahashi et al., 2012)
78 (Revenig et al., 2014)
79 (Koraitim, 2008)
80 (Patel et al., 2021)

Cohen, D., Gonzalez, J., & Goldstein, I. (2016). The role of pelvic floor muscles in male sexual dysfunction and pelvic pain. *Sexual Medicine Reviews, 4*(1), 53–62. https://doi.org/10.1016/j.sxmr.2015.10.001

Creed, K.E. (1995). Innervation of the smooth muscle of the lower urinary tract. *Journal of Smooth Muscle Research [Nihon Heikatsukin Gakkai Kikanshi], 31*(1), 1–4. https://doi.org/10.1540/jsmr.31.1

de Groat, W.C. (2006). Integrative control of the lower urinary tract: Preclinical perspective. *British Journal of Pharmacology, 147,* Suppl 2, S25–S40. https://doi.org/10.1038/sj.bjp.0706604

Dean, R.C., & Lue, T.F. (2005). Physiology of penile erection and pathophysiology of erectile dysfunction. *Urologic Clinics of North America, 32*(4), 379–395, v. https://doi.org/10.1016/j.ucl.2005.08.007

Dickinson, R. (1889). Studies of the levator ani muscle. *American Journal of Obstetrics and Diseases of Women and Children, 22*(9), 898–917.

Fine, S.W., & Reuter, V.E. (2012). Anatomy of the prostate revisited: Implications for prostate biopsy and zonal origins of prostate cancer. *Histopathology, 60*(1), 142–152. https://doi.org/10.1111/j.1365-2559.2011.04004.x

Frawley, H., Shelly, B., Morin, M., Bernard, S., *et al.* (2021). An International Continence Society (ICS) report on the terminology for pelvic floor muscle assessment. *Neurourology & Urodynamics, 40*(5), 1217–1260. https://doi.org/10.1002/nau.24658

Gray, H. (1988). *Gray's Anatomy: The Classic Collector's Edition* (Revised edition). Gramercy.

Hoeh, B., Wenzel, M., Hohenhorst, L., Köllermann, J., *et al.* (2022). Anatomical fundamentals and current surgical knowledge of prostate anatomy related to functional and oncological outcomes for robotic-assisted radical prostatectomy. *Frontiers in Surgery, 8,* 825183. https://doi.org/10.3389/fsurg.2021.825183

Hsu, G.-L. (2006). Hypothesis of human penile anatomy, erection hemodynamics and their clinical applications. *Asian Journal of Andrology, 8*(2), 225–234. https://doi.org/10.1111/j.1745-7262.2006.00108.x

Hsu, G.-L., Hsieh, C.-H., Wen, H.-S., Hsu, W.-L., *et al.* (2004). Anatomy of the human penis: The relationship of the architecture between skeletal and smooth muscles. *Journal of Andrology, 25*(3), 426–431. https://doi.org/10.1002/j.1939-4640.2004.tb02810.x

Koraitim, M.M. (2008). The male urethral sphincter complex revisited: An anatomical concept and its physiological correlate. *Journal of Urology, 179*(5), 1683–1689. https://doi.org/10.1016/j.juro.2008.01.010

Kumagai, S., Muraki, O., & Yoshimura, Y. (2022). Evaluation of the effect of levator ani muscle contraction on post-prostatectomy urinary incontinence using cine MRI. *Neurourology and Urodynamics, 41*(2), 616–625. https://doi.org/10.1002/nau.24861

Lindquist, C.M., Nikolaidis, P., Mittal, P.K., & Miller, F.H. (2020). MRI of the penis. *Abdominal Radiology, 45*(7), 2001–2017. https://doi.org/10.1007/s00261-019-02301-y

Mangera, A., Osman, N.I., & Chapple, C.R. (2013). Anatomy of the lower urinary tract. *Surgery – Oxford International Edition, 31*(7), 319–325. https://doi.org/10.1016/j.mpsur.2013.04.013

Patel, K., Mei, L., Yu, E., Kern, M., *et al.* (2021). Differences in fatigability of muscles involved in fecal continence: Potential clinical ramifications. *Physiological Reports, 9*(24), e15144. https://doi.org/10.14814/phy2.15144

Plochocki, J.H., Rodriguez-Sosa, J.R., Adrian, B., Ruiz, S.A., & Hall, M.I. (2016). A functional and clinical reinterpretation of human perineal neuromuscular anatomy: Application to sexual function and continence. *Clinical Anatomy (New York, N.Y.), 29*(8), 1053–1058. https://doi.org/10.1002/ca.22774

Ratanapornsompong, W., Pacharatakul, S., Sangkum, P., Leenanupan, C., & Kongcharoensombat, W. (2021). Effect of puboprostatic ligament preservation during robotic-assisted laparoscopic radical prostatectomy on early continence: Randomized controlled trial. *Asian Journal of Urology, 8*(3), 260. https://doi.org/10.1016/j.ajur.2020.11.002

Raychaudhuri, B., & Cahill, D. (2008). Pelvic fasciae in urology. *Annals of The Royal College of Surgeons of England, 90*(8), 633–637. https://doi.org/10.1308/003588408X321611

Rehder, P., Staudacher, N.M., Schachtner, J., Berger, M.E., *et al.* (2016). Hypothesis that urethral bulb (corpus spongiosum) plays an active role in male urinary continence. *Advances in Urology, 2016*, 6054730. https://doi.org/10.1155/2016/6054730

Revenig, L., Leung, A., & Hsiao, W. (2014). Ejaculatory physiology and pathophysiology: Assessment and treatment in male infertility. *Translational Andrology and Urology, 3*(1), 41–49. https://doi.org/10.3978/j.issn.2223-4683.2014.02.02

Rosier, P.F, de Wildt, M.J., de la Rosette, J.J., Debruyne, F.M., & Wijkstra, H. (1995). Analysis of maximum detrusor contraction power in relation to bladder emptying in patients with lower urinary tract symptoms and benign prostatic enlargement. *Journal of Urology, 154*(6), 2137–2142. https://doi.org/10.1016/S0022-5347(01)66716-8

Shobeiri, S.A., Chesson, R., & Gasser, R. (2008). The internal innervation and morphology of the human female levator ani muscle. *American Journal of Obstetrics and Gynecology, 199*, 686.e1-6. https://doi.org/10.1016/j.ajog.2008.07.057

Siccardi, M.A., & Bordoni, B. (2022). Anatomy, Abdomen and Pelvis, Perineal Body. In *StatPearls*. StatPearls Publishing. http://www.ncbi.nlm.nih.gov/books/NBK537345/

Sklinda, K., Frączek, M., Mruk, B., & Walecki, J. (2019). Normal 3T MR anatomy of the prostate gland and surrounding structures. *Advances in Medicine, 2019*, 3040859. https://doi.org/10.1155/2019/3040859

Stafford, R.E., Ashton-Miller, J.A., Constantinou, C.E., & Hodges, P.W. (2012). Novel insight into the dynamics of male pelvic floor contractions through transperineal ultrasound imaging. *Journal of Urology, 188*(4), 1224–1230. https://doi.org/10.1016/j.juro.2012.06.028

Stafford, R.E., Mazzone, S., Ashton-Miller, J.A., Constantinou, C., & Hodges, P.W. (2014). Dynamics of male pelvic floor muscle contraction observed with transperineal ultrasound imaging differ between voluntary and evoked coughs. *Journal of Applied Physiology (Bethesda, Md.: 1985), 116*(8), 953–960. https://doi.org/10.1152/japplphysiol.01225.2013

Suriyut, J., Muro, S., Baramee, P., Harada, M., & Akita, K. (2020). Various significant connections of the male pelvic floor muscles with special reference to the anal and urethral sphincter muscles. *Anatomical Science International, 95*(3), 305–312. https://doi.org/10.1007/s12565-019-00521-2

Tai, J.W., Sorkhi, S.R., Trivedi, I., Sakamoto, K., Albo, M., Bhargava, V., & Rajasekaran, M.R. (2021). Evaluation of age- and radical-prostatectomy related changes in male pelvic floor anatomy based on Magnetic Resonance Imaging and 3-Dimensional Reconstruction. *World Journal of Men's Health, 39*(3), 566. https://doi.org/10.5534/wjmh.200021

Talasz, H., Kremser, C., Talasz, H.J., Kofler, M., & Rudisch, A. (2022). Breathing, (s)training and the pelvic floor—A basic concept. *Healthcare, 10*(6), 1035. https://doi.org/10.3390/healthcare10061035

Tanahashi, M., Karicheti, V., Thor, K.B., & Marson, L. (2012). Characterization of bulbospongiosus muscle reflexes activated by urethral distension in male rats. *American Journal of Physiology–Regulatory, Integrative and Comparative Physiology, 303*(7), R737–R747. https://doi.org/10.1152/ajpregu.00004.2012

Wu, Y., Hikspoors, J.P.J.M., Mommen, G., Dabhoiwala, N.F., *et al.* (2020). Interactive three-dimensional teaching models of the female and male pelvic floor. *Clinical Anatomy (New York, N.Y.), 33*(2), 275–285. https://doi.org/10.1002/ca.23508

Yalla, S.V., Dibenedetto, M., Fam, B.A., Blunt, K.J., Constantinople, N., & Gabilondo, F.B. (1979). Striated sphincter participation in distal passive urinary continence mechanisms: Studies in male subjects deprived of proximal sphincter mechanism. *Journal of Urology, 122*(5), 655–660. https://doi.org/10.1016/s0022-5347(17)56546-5

CHAPTER 3

Tissue Modification After Radical Prostatectomy and Radiation Therapy

This chapter outlines the possible tissue changes and functional adaptations that may contribute to the side-effects of radical prostatectomy (RP) surgery and radiation. RP and radiation therapy can lead to a range of tissue changes, including scarring, nerve damage, inflammation, and fibrosis, which can result in side-effects such as urinary incontinence, erectile dysfunction, and bowel problems. Identifying these tissue modifications and adaptations resulting from treatments can help physiotherapists and healthcare providers predict and manage potential complications more effectively, providing patients with more personalized care. This approach may improve patients' quality of life and overall satisfaction with their treatment experience.

ANATOMY AND FUNCTIONAL CHANGES AFTER RADICAL PROSTATECTOMY

There are various anatomical and physiological theories that attempt to explain why men experience incontinence and erectile dysfunction following radical prostatectomy surgery. Even surgeons who have conducted numerous surgeries are uncertain why some men recover more quickly than others and why a small percentage of men continue to experience leakage even years after the surgery. The following section describes anatomical changes that occur after the surgery, which may lead to a decrease in urinary control and sexual function.

During RP the prostate is removed, along with the seminal vesicles, and the urethra is reconstructed via anastomosis of the membranous urethra to the bladder. The bladder is dropped to the area where the external urethral sphincter (EUS) is located which is then supported by the pelvic floor.[1] The bladder neck is "stretched" to fill the void of the prostate; the urethra support

---

1   (Kadono *et al.*, 2022)

system is altered and part of the internal urethral sphincter is removed (especially at the area of the bladder neck). The smooth muscles of the urethra may be compromised, especially if the neurovascular bundle of the prostate and the hypogastric nerve is removed or damaged.[2] There may be further operative complications such as severance to the supporting ligaments and fascia or damage to the external urethral sphincter or its nerves.[3] As a result of all these changes, even during reduced physical activities, urine passage may be facilitated by a bladder operating at high pressure, in a changed environment with decreased obstacles.[4]

Other studies have demonstrated reduced maximum urethral closure pressures and decreased striated urethral sphincter tonus after RP, and that the increase of maximal urethral closure pressure further along into recovery may be correlated to gaining urinary control.[5, 6] It was also proposed that after radical prostatectomy the urogenital diaphragm, which compresses the urethra from the outside, has to be in the proper position for maximum urethral pressure to occur.[7] Anatomical changes post-op, such as an upward shift (proximal) of the membranous urethra early post-op,[8] may shift this optimal position, changing and decreasing the urethral pressure (see Figure 3.1).

Bladder overactivity and decreased compliance was also noted post radical prostatectomy and could also contribute to voiding dysfunction after surgery.[9] Reduced bladder compliance can persist in 26% of cases eight months post RP, and bladder overactivity in 7–77% of patients after radical prostatectomy.[10] Reduced bladder compliance after RP may be due to direct injury to the trigone, bladder neck, or the urethral nerves, causing outlet incompetence and partial detrusor muscle denervation.[11] The reason for bladder overactivity after radical prostatectomy is unknown. In some cases, bladder overactivity may be presented before the surgery due to obstructive outlet syndrome, which can then be carried over after the surgery. Responses to inflammation, change and decrease of bladder support, and/or irritation due to catheterization may be possible causes of detrusor overactivity initiated post-surgery.

Another common form of urinary dysfunction post-RP is decreased urinary control with increased intra-abdominal pressure, termed as stress urinary incontinence (SUI). The external urethral sphincter and the levator ani

---

2   (Hoeh *et al.*, 2022)
3   (Heesakkers *et al.*, 2017)
4   (Abelson *et al.*, 2018)
5   (Yalla *et al.*, 1979)
6   (Dubbelman *et al.*, 2012)
7   (Kadono *et al.*, 2018)
8   (Kadono *et al.*, 2018)
9   (Porena *et al.*, 2007)
10 (Porena *et al.*, 2007)
11 (Porena *et al.*, 2007)

muscles contract in response to increased intra-abdominal pressure, the EUS compressing the urethra in an anterior–posterior direction, while the levator ani approximates the rectum towards the pubic bone in a posterior–anterior direction[12] (see Figure 3.2). After radical prostatectomy surgery it has been noted that the rectum may move less toward the pubic bone than before the surgery (especially on those individuals with urinary incontinence), which may decrease the pressure around the urethra and consequently increase the chances of SUI.[13] A recent study by Stafford et al. demonstrated through transperineal real time ultrasound that incontinent men post-radical prostatectomy had decreased displacement of the puborectalis, bulbocavernosus, and striated urinary sphincter during voluntary pelvic floor muscle contraction.[14]

Penile length changes have also been reported post-radical prostatectomy. The immediate pull on the cavernous tissue in a pelvic direction that can happen after vesicourethral anastomosis, and direct injury to the cavernous nerve causing hypoxia, were some of the reasons proposed for penile shortening post-radical prostatectomy.[15] Penile shortening can decrease passive urethral resistance and may affect passive urinary control.

Injury and removal of the neurovascular bundle and the arterial supply to the penis can also contribute to erectile dysfunction.[16, 17] Erectile dysfunction will be discussed in greater detail in Chapters 4 and 10.

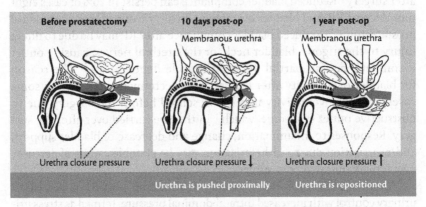

FIGURE 3.1: AN ILLUSTRATION OF URETHRAL CLOSURE PRESSURE
AND MEMBRANOUS URETHRA CHANGES AFTER RP
Adapted and modified from Kadono et al., 2018[18]

12 (Stafford et al., 2012)
13 (Kumagai et al., 2022)
14 (Stafford et al., 2020)
15 (Kadono et al., 2022)
16 (Magheli & Burnett, 2009)
17 (Hoeh et al., 2022)
18 (Kadono et al., 2018)

Pre-radical prostatectomy

Post-radical prostatectomy

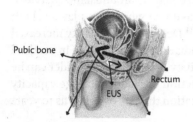

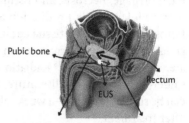

| EUS contraction direction and displacement with increased intra-abdominal pressure | Levator ani contraction direction and displacement with increased intra-abdominal pressure | EUS contraction direction and displacement with increased intra-abdominal pressure | Levator ani contraction direction and displacement with increased intra-abdominal pressure |

FIGURE 3.2: THEORETICAL REPRESENTATION OF
URETHRAL COMPRESSION PRE AND POST RP
Image owned by Samantha Hughes, all rights reserved

PHYSIOLOGICAL AND FUNCTIONAL CHANGES AFTER RADIATION THERAPY

As described in Chapter 1, radiation therapy (RT) destroys and damages cancer DNA cells via high energy rays. Newer technological advancements and the use of intensity-modulated radiation therapy techniques have been more successful in increasing the dosage to the targeted area while decreasing the radiation effects to the bladder and rectum.[19] However, tissue changes in the bladder and rectum can still occur, affecting the healthy tissues temporarily and sometimes permanently. With each exposure to RT, micro-lesions can occur to healthy tissue, promoting an inflammatory response for every fraction delivered, affecting tissue which is already going through cellular repair, inflammation, or injury.[20] In other words, the wound healing process that happens with radiation differs from other traumatic wound healing because of the accumulating and repetitive nature of it, and because wound healing is happening during the entire course of RT sessions, repairing "normal" tissue which will look very different in nature from the first few radiation sessions compared to the last sessions.

The radiation-induced lesions to bladder and rectal tissues occur due to a complex interaction of processes including the alterations of cellular and extracellular components, progressive changes of the extracellular matrix, and vascular responses.[21, 22] Extracellular-connective-tissue stroma

---

19 (Martin & D'Amico, 2014)
20 (Denham & Hauer-Jensen, 2002)
21 (Denham & Hauer-Jensen, 2002)
22 (Baker & Krochak, 1989)

cell (e.g., fibroblast) degradation can also occur and may be associated with haemorrhage, necrosis, and fistula.[23] There may be an imbalance between extracellular matrix production and breakdown which can play a role in fibrosis and decreased tissue compliance.[24] Decreased vascularity increased collagen density and organization after radiation can play a role in urethral stenosis and strictures.[25] Radiation sensitivity of the urinary bladder can be underestimated in the literature, as reduction of bladder storage capacity can be seen as soon as 3–4 weeks after radiation therapy or as late as 10 years after treatment.[26]

RT can also be linked to promoting damage to the rectal mucosa, to increasing rectal sensitivity, and reducing anal resting pressure.[27] It may be hypothesized that RT may damage the internal anal sphincter nerve supply, causing passive fecal incontinence in some individuals.[28] Consequently, all these changes after radiation treatments can affect bladder and bowel function, making their stretch receptors more sensitive to volume changes and increasing the risk for developing painful urination, urgency, frequency, and incontinence of urine and feces. More on the side-effects of radiation treatment will be discussed in Chapter 4.

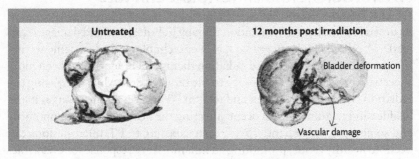

FIGURE 3.3: EXAMPLE OF MICE BLADDER DEFORMITY
AND VASCULAR CHANGES AFTER RADIATION
Image modified from Zwaans et al., 2020.[29]

CONCLUSION

Understanding the anatomical, physiological, and cellular changes that happen after radical prostatectomy and radiation treatment gives patients, family members, and clinicians a broader view of possible reasons why and how

23   (Streltsova *et al.*, 2021)
24   (Herrera *et al.*, 2018)
25   (Hughes *et al.*, 2020)
26   (Jaal *et al.*, 2004)
27   (Petersen *et al.*, 2014)
28   (Petersen *et al.*, 2014)
29   (Zwaans *et al.*, 2020)

these treatments impact prostate cancer survivors. The profound anatomical changes after radical prostatectomy and tissue alterations after radiation therapy can affect sexual, bladder, and bowel function in the acute and chronic phases of healing. However, these theoretical physiological explanations for the side-effect of prostate cancer treatments can only *partially* justify post-treatment impairments, as treatments will not have the same effect in every prostate cancer patient. Fortunately, some individuals will have few side-effects for a short period of time, but most unfortunately, others will have significant life-altering symptoms which may impact the rest of their lives.

REFERENCES

Abelson, B., Sun, D., Que, L., Nebel, R.A., et al. (2018). Sex differences in lower urinary tract biology and physiology. *Biology of Sex Differences, 9*(1), 45. https://doi.org/10.1186/s13293-018-0204-8

Baker, D.G., & Krochak, R J. (1989). The response of the microvascular system to radiation: A review. *Cancer Investigation, 7*(3), 287–294. https://doi.org/10.3109/07357908909039849

Denham, J.W., & Hauer-Jensen, M. (2002). The radiotherapeutic injury—A complex 'wound.' *Radiotherapy and Oncology, 63*(2), 129–145. https://doi.org/10.1016/S0167-8140(02)00060-9

Dubbelman, Y.D., Groen, J., Wildhagen, M.F., Rikken, B., & Bosch, J.L.H.R. (2012). Urodynamic quantification of decrease in sphincter function after radical prostatectomy: Relation to postoperative continence status and the effect of intensive pelvic floor muscle exercises. *Neurourology and Urodynamics, 31*(5), 646–651. https://doi.org/10.1002/nau.21243

Heesakkers, J., Farag, F., Bauer, R.M., Sandhu, J., De Ridder, D., & Stenzl, A. (2017). Pathophysiology and contributing factors in postprostatectomy incontinence: A review. *European Urology, 71*(6), 936–944. https://doi.org/10.1016/j.eururo.2016.09.031

Herrera, J., Henke, C.A., & Bitterman, P.B. (2018). Extracellular matrix as a driver of progressive fibrosis. *Journal of Clinical Investigation, 128*(1), 45–53. https://doi.org/10.1172/JCI93557

Hoeh, B., Wenzel, M., Hohenhorst, L., Köllermann, J., et al. (2022). Anatomical fundamentals and current surgical knowledge of prostate anatomy related to functional and oncological outcomes for robotic-assisted radical prostatectomy. *Frontiers in Surgery, 8*, 825183. https://doi.org/10.3389/fsurg.2021.825183

Hughes, M., Caza, T., Li, G., Daugherty, M., Blakley, S., & Nikolavsky, D. (2020). Histologic characterization of the post-radiation urethral stenosis in men treated for prostate cancer. *World Journal of Urology, 38*(9), 2269–2277. https://doi.org/10.1007/s00345-019-03031-y

Kadono, Y., Nohara, T., Kawaguchi, S., Iwamoto, H., et al. (2022). Impact of pelvic anatomical changes caused by radical prostatectomy. *Cancers, 14*(13), Article 13. https://doi.org/10.3390/cancers14133050

Kadono, Y., Nohara, T., Kawaguchi, S., Naito, R., et al. (2018). Investigating the mechanism underlying urinary continence recovery after radical prostatectomy: Effectiveness of a longer urethral stump to prevent urinary incontinence. *BJU International, 122*(3), 456–462. https://doi.org/10.1111/bju.14181

Jaal, J., Brüchner, K., Hoinkis, C., & Dörr, W. (2004). Radiation-induced variations in urothelial expression of intercellular adhesion molecule 1 (ICAM-1): Association with changes in urinary bladder function. *International Journal of Radiation Biology, 80*(1), 65–72. https://doi.org/10.1080/09553000310001632921

Kumagai, S., Muraki, O., & Yoshimura, Y. (2022). Evaluation of the effect of levator ani muscle contraction on post-prostatectomy urinary incontinence using cine MRI. *Neurourology and Urodynamics, 41*(2), 616–625. https://doi.org/10.1002/nau.24861

Magheli, A., & Burnett, A.L. (2009). Erectile dysfunction following prostatectomy: Prevention and treatment. *Nature Reviews Urology, 6*(8), Article 8. https://doi.org/10.1038/nrurol.2009.126

Martin, N.E., & D'Amico, A.V. (2014). Progress and controversies: Radiation therapy for prostate cancer. *CA: A Cancer Journal for Clinicians, 64*(6), 389–407. https://doi.org/10.3322/caac.21250

Petersen, S.E., Høyer, M., Bregendahl, S., Laurberg, S., *et al.* (2014). Pathophysiology of late anorectal dysfunction following external beam radiotherapy for prostate cancer. *Acta Oncologica, 53*(10), 1398–1404. https://doi.org/10.3109/0284186X.2014.926029

Porena, M., Mearini, E., Mearini, L., Vianello, A., & Giannantoni, A. (2007). Voiding dysfunction after radical retropubic prostatectomy: More than external urethral sphincter deficiency. *European Urology, 52*(1), 38–45. https://doi.org/10.1016/j.eururo.2007.03.051

Stafford, R.E., Ashton-Miller, J.A., Constantinou, C.E., & Hodges, P.W. (2012). Novel insight into the dynamics of male pelvic floor contractions through transperineal ultrasound imaging. *Journal of Urology, 188*(4), 1224–1230. https://doi.org/10.1016/j.juro.2012.06.028

Stafford, R.E., Coughlin, G., & Hodges, P.W. (2020). Comparison of dynamic features of pelvic floor muscle contraction between men with and without incontinence after prostatectomy and men with no history of prostate cancer. *Neurourology and Urodynamics, 39*(1), 170–180. https://doi.org/10.1002/nau.24213

Streltsova, O., Kiseleva, E., Dudenkova, V., Sergeeva, E., *et al.* (2021). Late changes in the extracellular matrix of the bladder after radiation therapy for pelvic tumors. *Diagnostics, 11*(9), Article 9. https://doi.org/10.3390/diagnostics11091615

Yalla, S.V., Dibenedetto, M., Fam, B.A., Blunt, K.J., Constantinople, N., & Gabilondo, F.B. (1979). Striated sphincter participation in distal passive urinary continence mechanisms: Studies in male subjects deprived of proximal sphincter mechanism. *Journal of Urology, 122*(5), 655–660. https://doi.org/10.1016/s0022-5347(17)56546-5

Zwaans, B.M.M., Wegner, K.A., Bartolone, S.N., Vezina, C.M., Chancellor, M.B., & Lamb, L.E. (2020). Radiation cystitis modeling: A comparative study of bladder fibrosis radio-sensitivity in C57BL/6, C3H, and BALB/c mice. *Physiological Reports, 8*(4), e14377. https://doi.org/10.14814/phy2.14377

CHAPTER 4

Side-Effects of Prostate Cancer and Treatments

The side-effects of prostate cancer and its treatments can significantly impact the lives of men and their families. Ongoing psychological, physical, emotional, social, informational, and sexual support is often needed for those diagnosed with prostate cancer and undergoing treatment, depending on the stage of cancer and treatments received. It's important to note that treatments can be given in isolation or in combination, and side-effects may accumulate over time. Symptoms such as pain and urinary, bowel, and sexual dysfunction can arise soon after treatment or years later.

This chapter aims to discuss the most common symptoms and side-effects of prostate cancer and its treatments, as well as proposed pathophysiology, to help physiotherapists and health professionals better tailor their approaches, treatments, and programs for their patients.

URINARY INCONTINENCE

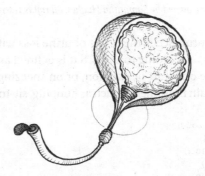

Urinary incontinence (UI) is defined by the International Continence Society (ICS) as the complaint of urinary loss. Most specifically, UI can be categorized into stress urinary incontinence (SUI) and urge urinary incontinence. Mixed

UI is a term used for individuals presented with both types of UI. Other types of UI relevant to prostate cancer survivors include climacturia (urine loss during sexual climax or orgasm), and post-void dribbles (urinary leakage after urination).

Urinary incontinence is one of the most common side-effects of prostate cancer treatment. Prevalence of UI post cancer treatments varies significantly (ranging from 66% to 20%),[1, 2] and is probably due to a lack of a consistent definition and quantifiable measurement of UI in the studies.[3] Post-prostatectomy urinary incontinence (PPUI) can be long term in 20–33% of men post-prostatectomy,[4, 5, 6] and UI can be present in 10–15% post external beam radiation[7] one year after treatment.

UI can significantly impact men's quality of life, increase the risk of institutionalization in older men,[8] and be a risk factor for depression and anxiety.[9] Men with UI can also have poorer self-perceived general health compared to men who are continent.[10]

Stress urinary incontinence

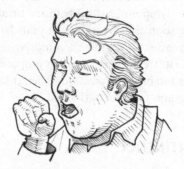

Image owned by Samantha Hughes, all rights reserved

Stress urinary incontinence is the result of urine loss with increased intra-abdominal pressure. According to the ICS it is defined as "the complaint of involuntary leakage on effort or exertion, or on sneezing or coughing."[11] It can occur with certain movements (such as jumping, sit-to-stand, or bending

1   (Katz & Rodriguez, 2007)
2   (Ficarra *et al.*, 2012)
3   (Wilson & Gilling, 2011)
4   (Nilsson *et al.*, 2011)
5   (Wei & Montie, 2000)
6   (Tienza *et al.*, 2018)
7   (Liu *et al.*, 2005)
8   (Baztan, 2005)
9   (Felde *et al.*, 2017)
10 (Kwong *et al.*, 2010)
11 (Abrams *et al.*, 2002)

down), lifting, or laughing. Stress urinary incontinence is of short duration and can only happen intermittently.[12] Prostatectomy surgery is the most common cause for SUI in men,[13] and it is commonly more profound right after surgery, improving with time, with a large number of men recovering continence at 6–12 months post-op.[14] The pathophysiology of SUI in men post-prostatectomy could be mostly attributed to sphincteric deficiency, as maximal urethral closure pressure appears to be reduced after surgery.[15] It is hypothesized that the cause for sphincteric deficiency post-prostatectomy is mostly due to temporary nerve damage or change to the structural support to the external urethral sphincter rather than a direct injury to it, as recovery usually improves over time.[16]

These are the main predictors for post-prostatectomy urinary incontinence reported in the literature:[17, 18]

- the amount of leakage post-catheter removal can be a strong predictive factor of regaining urinary continence post-prostatectomy; for example, men who have less than 10% urine loss at the day of catheter removal can have higher chances of being dry three months post-op
- *age; the older the individual the more likely is development of SUI post-surgery
- pre-operative length of membranous urethra
- body mass index
- stages of disease
- prior transurethral resection of the prostate (TURP)
- *low level of education
- *salvage radiation therapy
- *respiratory disease
- surgeon's experience.

* There are strong predictors for long-term UI post-prostatectomy.

Urge urinary incontinence and overactive bladder

Urge incontinence is the complaint of involuntary leakage accompanied by or immediately preceded by urgency (ICS).[19] Overactive bladder (OAB) syndrome consists of urinary urgency, and frequent urination with or without

---

12 (Yalla *et al.*, 1982)
13 (Groutz *et al.*, 2000)
14 (Das *et al.*, 2020)
15 (Hoyland *et al.*, 2014)
16 (Hoyland *et al.*, 2014)
17 (Tatenuma *et al.*, 2021)
18 (Nilsson *et al.*, 2011)
19 (Abrams *et al.*, 2002)

urgency incontinence.[20] With an overactive bladder, the sensation to urinate, which will usually happen when the bladder is about half-full, will happen much sooner, consequently increasing urination frequency at much smaller volumes. Occasionally, the strong sensation to urinate may cause urinary leakages, and this fear or leaking can result in detrimental coping behaviors, such as being preoccupied with knowing where every toilet is or avoiding activities and participation.

OAB may present with decreased bladder compliance and hyper-excitability of the detrusor muscles. These changes in the bladder physiology may be attributed to decreased maximum urethral closure pressure post-prostatectomy,[21] denervation and devascularization of the bladder, or inflammatory changes related to the surgery.[22] According to urodynamics studies, detrusor dysfunction—including poor compliance and detrusor overactivity—can be commonly seen post-prostatectomy with incidence ranging over 20–40%.[23, 24]

In radiation therapy patients, OAB could be associated with cellular and tissue changes (as discussed in Chapter 3) causing detrusor instability or obstructive outlet.[25, 26] Following prostate cancer treatments, brachytherapy results in higher incidence of OAB syndrome compared to surgery and external beam radiation therapy.[27] Factors that can influence OAB and urgency incontinence include the following:

- Arteriosclerosis may be a predictor for the development of OAB post-prostatectomy.[28]
- Anxiety and depression can be linked to symptoms of OAB, or it may be a causation factor for OAB.[29, 30]
- Previous lower urinary tract symptoms (LUTS) before prostate cancer treatment can also be a predictor for OAB and urgency UI after prostate cancer treatments.[31]

20   (Abrams et al., 2003)
21   (Lee & Lee, 2021)
22   (Hoyland et al., 2014)
23   (Leach et al., 1996)
24   (Kielb & Clemens, 2005)
25   (Denham & Hauer-Jensen, 2002)
26   (Khan et al., 2021)
27   (Khan et al., 2021)
28   (Koguchi et al., 2019)
29   (Melotti et al., 2018)
30   (Lai et al., 2016)
31   (Pastore et al., 2017)

POST-PROSTATECTOMY PASSIVE URINARY INCONTINENCE

Clinically, when you assess and treat UI post-prostatectomy, you may note a large number of cases where UI happens inexplicably and without awareness, or, more severely, urine will passively dribble out (like a faucet/tap not properly closed) while in a standing position (gravitational incontinence). These types of UI can be further classified as *passive UI*. Yalla and colleagues' urodynamics study demonstrated that 13/21 subjects had passive incontinence post-prostatectomy and three of those had gravitational incontinence. The one subject with severe gravitational incontinence presented with periurethral denervation but normal detrusor contractions.[32] This loss of urine happening randomly at low pressure and without the sense of urgency or detrusor contraction can theoretically be contributed by weakening or damage to the smooth sphincter muscles or decreased resting tone of the striated sphincter.[33] This can result in decreased urine accumulation in the bladder, where in some cases, the perception to urinate is absent.

According to Professor Wilhelm Hubner's latest ICS2022 presentation, passive UI may be the most common type of leakage post-prostatectomy, possibly due to damage or removal of the hypogastric nerve contained in the neurovascular bundle of the prostate.[34] He further suggested that the striated sphincter usually is intact as the pudendal nerve is not commonly affected during surgery.

Post-void dribbling

Post-void dribbling is a type of urine leakage which usually happens after urination. A few drops of urine will come out as soon as the individual finishes urinating. It is commonly seen in males post-prostatectomy and there is also an association between post-void dribbling and urge incontinence.[35] The theory proposed for post-void dribbling after prostatectomy surgery is that, after the surgery, the urine is trapped in the penile or bulbar urethra (maybe due to structural changes after anastomosis), and it begins to leak out as soon as urination finishes but stops once the urethra is completely drained.[36]

32 (Yalla *et al.*, 1982)
33 (Yalla *et al.*, 1979)
34 (ICS 2022, n.d.)
35 (Ablove, 2010)
36 (Nickel & Speakman, 2019)

Climacturia

Climacturia is the complaint of involuntary loss of urine at the time of orgasm, as defined by the ICS.[37] It is quite prevalent after prostate cancer treatments, especially post-prostatectomy.[38, 39] There may be an association between climacturia and stress urinary incontinence, orgasmic pain, and penile shortening in those after prostatectomy.[40] There is also a strong relationship with climacturia and those who use aids to obtain an erection.[41] The pathophysiology of climacturia after prostatectomy surgery has yet to be appropriately tested, but a few proposed mechanisms were reported:[42]

- penile shortening due to cavernous nerve injury, and change to the corpora cavernosa smooth muscle tone due to an increased sympathetic drive, possibly having an effect on the length of the intrinsic urethral sphincter
- removal of the internal urethral sphincter and external urethral sphincter relaxation at the time of orgasm
- bladder neck spasms occurring at the vesicourethral anastomosis resulting in orgasmic pain, which can influence climacturia
- bladder detrusor contraction at the time of orgasm with external sphincter relaxation.

RADIATION CYSTITIS

Radiation cystitis is a term used to define inflammatory and tissue changes to the bladder—promoting lower urinary tract symptoms, such as burning with urination, frequency, urgency, bleeding, and decreased bladder capacity—following radiation therapy to the pelvic organs. These symptoms can be presented during the acute phase, occurring up to or during three months of completion of treatment, and/or in late phases of radiation, which typically occur after 2–3 years of treatment completion, but it can even occur after 10 years of treatment.[43] The severity of symptoms can vary from microscopic hematuria (blood with urination) with mild lower urinary tract symptoms, to severe symptoms with gross hematuria, urinary incontinence, blood clot, and, on rare occasions, death.[44] The Franco-Italian and the LENT-SOMA are the two common grading systems for radiation cystitis symptom severity classification (Figures 4.1 and 4.2).

---

37   (Kocjancic *et al.*, 2022)
38   (Salter, 2020)
39   (O'Neil *et al.*, 2014)
40   (Choi *et al.*, 2007)
41   (O'Neil *et al.*, 2014)
42   (Kannady & Clavell Hernandez, 2020)
43   (Helissey *et al.*, 2020)
44   (Murphy *et al.*, 2019)

Acute radiation cystitis is mostly due to an acute inflammatory response and tissue edema as a result of post-radiation injury to the bladder mucosa.[45] It can affect about 50% of localized prostate cancer patients receiving radiation therapy. In most cases, symptoms will subside 4–6 weeks following treatment.[46]

Late radiation hemorrhagic cystitis can be the response of histological tissue change (as mentioned in Chapter 3) causing ulceration and mal formed blood vessels which are fragile and prone to bleeding.[47] Its incidence rate has been reported to be in between 5% and 10% in patients receiving prostate cancer radiation therapy[48]—being higher after receiving external beam radiation and intensity-modulated radiation therapy, and the lowest after brachytherapy.[49] Late radiation cystitis response risks are multifactorial and can include:[50, 51]

- Pre-existing medical conditions such as hypertension and diabetes
- Tumor extent
- Precise radiation details such as volume treated, total bladder dose, and rate of treatment
- Concurrent treatments such as chemotherapy or surgery
- Genetic predisposition.

GRADE 0	No symptoms
GRADE 1 Mild complications	Mild symptoms lasting < 6 months, residual volume less than 100 cc, mild hematuria, minor incontinence
GRADE 2 Moderate complications	Hematuria requiring hospitalization, postural incontinence, symptoms lasting > 6 months, urethral stenosis requiring dilatation
GRADE 3 Severe complications	Severe hematuria requiring surgery, total incontinence, permanent bladder retention, urethral stenosis requiring surgery
GRADE 4	Death

FIGURE 4.1: FRANCO-ITALIAN GLOSSARY GRADING
SYSTEM FOR RADIATION CYSTITIS[52]

---

45 (Rigaud et al., 2004)
46 (Rigaud et al., 2004)
47 (Martin et al., 2019)
48 (Sanguedolce et al., 2021)
49 (Martin et al., 2019)
50 (Denton et al., 2002)
51 (Zwaans et al., 2020)
52 (Chassagne et al., 1993)

GRADE 0	No toxicity
GRADE 1	Minor symptoms that don't need treatment
GRADE 2	Symptoms needing conservative treatment
GRADE 3	Severe symptoms, impacting life tasks and requiring more aggressive treatment
GRADE 4	Irreversible functional damage needing major intervention
GRADE 5	Death or organ failure

FIGURE 4.2: LENT-SOMA GRADING SYSTEM[53]

FECAL INCONTINENCE

As defined by the ICS, fecal incontinence (FI) is the complaint of involuntary loss of feces—when solid and/or liquid.[54] With FI, feces discharge can happen involuntarily without the awareness to defecate, seep, or soil following normal evacuation, or can occur with strong urge to defecate without the ability to actively retain the fecal matter.[55] Rectal sensation, rectal compliance, and the ability to recognize the urge need to be intact in order to experience continence and normal evacuation.[56] Fecal incontinence is a known side-effect following radiation therapy, including external beam radiation, intensity modulated therapy, and brachytherapy, and it can affect up to 58% of prostate cancer radiation patients in the acute and latent phase of treatment.[57] FI can significantly impact quality of life, sexual involvement, and function.[58,59] There are very few published studies evaluating the potential mechanism for FI after radiotherapy. Some theories suggested that FI post-radiation could result from an injury to the nerve plexus of the rectal muscular layer, especially affecting the external anal sphincter. Fecal incontinence could also be the result of fibrotic changes to the rectum wall, which may cause reduced rectal capacity, urgency, and urge fecal incontinence.[60]

---

53 (Mornex *et al.*, 1997)
54 (D'Ancona *et al.*, 2019)
55 (Rao, 2004)
56 (Cash & Glass, 2016)
57 (Maeda *et al.*, 2011)
58 (Ouizeman *et al.*, 2020)
59 (Muñoz-Yagüe *et al.*, 2014)
60 (Maeda *et al.*, 2011)

ERECTILE DYSFUNCTION

According to ICS terminology, erectile dysfunction (ED) is the consistent or recurrent inability to attain and/or maintain a penile erection sufficient for sexual satisfaction and/or sexual intercourse.[61] Erectile dysfunction is one of the major complications after localized prostate cancer treatments, incidence rates ranging at 8–85% after radiation therapy and 26–100% after prostatectomy.[62] Sexual dysfunction in men can negatively impact their self-esteem, body image, and psychological health, increasing chances of depression and anxiety.[63] It has been proposed that temporary injury to the cavernous nerve during treatment (especially after prostate surgery), will cause penile hypoxia, smooth muscle cell death, fibrosis, and decreased venous occlusion, consequently affecting penile erection.[64] Age can also influence ED, as men over 60 years old have a lesser chance of erectile function recovery post radical prostatectomy, compared to men younger than 60 years old.[65] It could be estimated that a large number of men 60 years or older would be experiencing changes in the quality of erections even prior to prostate cancer treatments, as age is an independent risk factor for ED.[66] Nerve-sparing procedures can also improve erectile function recovery, especially after 18 months post radical prostatectomy.[67]

SIDE-EFFECTS FROM ANDROGEN DEPRIVATION THERAPY

Androgen deprivation therapy (ADT) is widely used independently or in conjunction with other forms of treatments, mostly for those with moderate to high risk and metastatic prostate cancer. ADT can induce debilitating effects, especially on those who have been using it for a long period of time. The relative risks for developing side-effects will be dependent on the type of drug used, the duration of treatment, and other comorbidities. The ADT side-effects identified in Edmunds and colleagues' systematic review[68] are discussed below.

Bone changes

Bone loss, osteoporosis, and bone fractures have been identified as possible risks for ADT treatment. The combination of ageing and ADT can further increase the chances for bone health deterioration. Furthermore, bone fracture can increase the rate of mortality to 40%.

---

61 (Kocjancic et al., 2022)
62 (Burnett et al., 2007)
63 (Twitchell et al., 2019)
64 (Magheli & Burnett, 2009)
65 (Tal et al., 2009)
66 (Mulhall et al., 2016)
67 (Tal et al., 2009)
68 (Edmunds et al., 2020)

Metabolic changes
Changes in body composition such as increase in body fat, decrease in lean mass, and increase in body mass index were identified after ADT, especially greater in the first three months of treatment. Furthermore, the risks of acquiring metabolic syndrome (increased waist circumference, alteration in lipids, and decreased insulin sensitivity) was 75% higher in prostate cancer patients receiving ADT compared to those who weren't. Prostate cancer patients receiving ADT can also have 39% higher risk for developing diabetes.

Cardiovascular changes
Certain ADT drugs may have a higher increased risk than others of cardiovascular changes and events, such as hypertension, myocardial infarction, stroke, deep vein thrombosis, and pulmonary embolism. Hot flashes or increased vasomotor flushing was also associated with ADT administered to prostate cancer patients in different disease stages or treatment combinations.

Sexual dysfunction
Decreased libido and erectile dysfunction are usually common complaints from ADT prostate cancer patients and their partners. Radiation therapy patients receiving a combination of short-term ADT had higher rates of sexual dysfunction at one-year post-treatment compared to those receiving radiation therapy alone.[69]

Depression
There may be an increased risk of developing depression for those prostate cancer survivors receiving intermittent or continuous ADT treatment.

Other changes
ADT can also increase the risk of falls, induce fatigue, and decrease body strength. These symptoms can be related to the type of ADT drugs, and decline in physical function can be most meaningful within 3–6 months of treatment.

CHEMOTHERAPY INDUCED PERIPHERAL NEUROPATHY
The most common type of chemotherapy drug prescribed to prostate cancer patients are taxane drugs (docetaxel and cabazitaxel).[70] Chemotherapy induced peripheral neuropathy (CIPN) is a common side-effect of taxane drugs, and can persist for several years in about 30% of patients receiving

69   (Jones *et al.*, 2011)
70   (Johns Hopkins Medicine, 2019)

them. Most commonly, the symptoms experienced from CIPN are sensory in nature and include tingling, numbness, and pain (dysesthesias, allodynia, hyperpathia) on the extremities. Motor changes such as muscle weakness, cramps, or gait dysfunction, and autonomic changes such as constipation/ diarrhoea, sweating abnormalities, and positional light-headedness or dizziness may also occur, although less frequently.[71] These sensorial changes and symptoms have an unacknowledged impact on quality of life and safety, for example, prostate cancer patients with CIPN have a three-fold increased risk of falls.[72]

The pathophysiology of this condition may be attributed to microtubule disruption altering axonal transport, in turn changing ion channel activity and leading to hyperexcitability of peripheral neurons. Other possible contributors of CIPN are mitochondrial damage leading to demyelination of peripheral nerves, altered expression of ion channels, and release of inflammatory cytokines due to activation of immune cells.[73]

Some predisposing factors were identified in the literature, including: age, pre-existing neuropathy (such as diabetic neuropathy), smoking, impaired renal function, exposure to other chemotherapy neurotoxic agents, and direct cancer-associated neuropathy.[74]

The American Society of Clinical Oncology recommends the use of the EORTC QLQ-CIPN20 questionnaire (Figure 4.3) as a tool to assess patients' experience of symptoms and functional limitations related to CIPN. However, its use in clinical settings may still be limited.[75]

71   (Ewertz et al., 2015)
72   (Kolb et al., 2016)
73   (Zajączkowska et al., 2019)
74   (Seretny et al., 2014)
75   (Mols et al., 2016)

EORTC QLQ – CIPN20

Patients sometimes report that they have the following symptoms or problems. Please indicate the extent to which you have experienced these symptoms or problems during the past week. Please answer by circling the number that best applies to you.

During the past week:	Not at All	A Little	Quite a Bit	Very Much
31 Did you have tingling fingers or hands?	1	2	2	4
32 Did you have tingling toes or feet?	1	2	2	4
33 Did you have numbness in your fingers or hands?	1	2	2	4
34 Did you have numbness in your toes or feet?	1	2	2	4
35 Did you have shooting or burning pain in your fingers or hands?	1	2	2	4
36 Did you have shooting or burning pain in your toes or feet?	1	2	2	4
37 Did you have cramps in your hands?	1	2	2	4
38 Did you have cramps in your feet?	1	2	2	4
39 Did you have problems standing or walking because of difficulty feeling the ground under your feet?	1	2	2	4
40 Did you have difficulty distinguishing between hot and cold water?	1	2	2	4
41 Did you have a problem holding a pen, which made writing difficult?	1	2	2	4
42 Did you have difficulty manipulating small objects with your fingers (for example, fastening small buttons)?	1	2	2	4
43 Did you have difficulty opening a jar or bottle because of weakness in your hands?	1	2	2	4
44 Did you have difficulty walking because your feet dropped downwards?	1	2	2	4
45 Did you have difficulty climbing stairs or getting up out of a chair because of weakness in your legs?	1	2	2	4
46 Were you dizzy when standing up from a sitting or lying position?	1	2	2	4
47 Did you have blurred vision?	1	2	2	4
48 Did you have difficulty hearing?	1	2	2	4

Please answer the following question only if you drive a car

	Not at All	A Little	Quite a Bit	Very Much
49 Did you have difficulty using the pedals?	1	2	2	4

Please answer the following question only if you are a man

	Not at All	A Little	Quite a Bit	Very Much
50 Did you have difficulty getting or maintaining an erection?	1	2	2	4

FIGURE 4.3: EORTC QLQ-CIPN20

CANCER-RELATED FATIGUE

Cancer-related fatigue (CRF) is a very common complaint in cancer care, and experienced in up to 74% of prostate cancer survivors. Fatigue can be experienced before, after, and during treatments (prostatectomy, ADT, chemo- and radiotherapy), or it can be perceived many years after treatment completion.[76] CRF can profoundly impact prostate cancer survivors' psychosocial status, interfering with work or everyday tasks, and may promote delay or termination of treatment.[77] The National Comprehensive Cancer Network (NCCN) in the USA described CRF as "a common, persistent, and subjective sense of tiredness related to cancer or to treatment for cancer that interferes with usual functioning."[78] Cancer-related fatigue is a more severe form of fatigue that is not relieved by rest and is usually found in combination with other side-effects of prostate cancer, such as pain, urinary symptoms, anxiety, depression, and sleep disturbance.[79]

The pathophysiology of CRF is poorly understood, and it is often complex and multifactorial. Many mechanisms were proposed to contribute to cancer-related fatigue, which can be directly related to the cancer or in combination with other phenomena indirectly related to the disease. Some of the proposed mechanisms or causes of CRF were:[80, 81]

- Anemia
- Stress
- Malnutrition
- Post-surgical fatigue
- Chemotherapy related fatigue proposed to be due to anemia, neurotoxicities, or accumulation of cell end product
- Radiotherapy related fatigue
- Infection
- Metabolic disorders, such as diabetes and cardiovascular diseases
- Psychosocial disorders, such as anxiety and depression
- Sleep disorders
- Hormonal changes
- Skeletal muscles changes.

---

76 (McConkey, 2016)
77 (McConkey, 2016)
78 (Mock, 2000)
79 (McConkey, 2016)
80 (Stasi et al., 2003)
81 (Gutstein, 2001)

PAIN

Pain, defined by the International Association for the Study of Pain (IASP), is "an unpleasant sensory and *emotional* experience associated with actual or *potential* tissue damage or described in terms of such damage"; the IASP also identifies pain as a *personal experience* influenced by *biological, psychological, and social factors,* and which cannot be inferred solely from activity in sensory neurons.[82]

Pain can greatly reduce cancer patients' health status, and can be a consequence directly related to tumor involvement, to diagnostic procedures, from the side-effects of treatment, or unrelated to any of these.[83] Pain is one of the most frequent persistent symptoms in cancer survivors.[84] Moderate to severe pain can be experienced in about 45–50% of curable cancer patients and over 70% of patients with advanced palliative cancer.[85] An average of about 60% of prostate cancer patients can experience pain, which is associated with increased disease burden and reduced quality of life.[86] Advanced prostate cancer (APC) pain is particularly common and mostly experienced by patients with bone metastatic disease, ranging from 47% to over 70%.[87, 88] APC pain can also be associated with psychological symptoms, such as fatigue, depression, and anxiety, reduced physical function, urinary and sexual dysfunction, and increased comorbidities.[89] Although prostate cancer patients with pain have an increased risk of having bone metastases, a direct relationship between the location of bone metastases and skeletal pain was not found in prostate cancer patients—for example: bone metastases in the same individual may produce pain in one skeletal area, but not in another. Furthermore, pain is often unassociated with the degree or size of bone involvement.[90] This illustrates the notion that cancer pain is a phenomenon influenced by many other factors beyond a localized tissue response, and that the type of cancer, or its size, does not necessarily predict symptoms.

Other specific types of prostate cancer survivors' pain can include radiation therapy induced painful urination (8.8%)[91] and taxane acute pain syndrome (TAPS) during taxane based chemotherapy (36.2%).[92] The latest is usually presented in a form of arthralgia (joint pain) and myalgia (muscle pain), starting one to three days after receiving the infusion and lasting for

---

82 (International Association for the Study of Pain, n.d.)
83 (Bader *et al.*, 2012)
84 (Nijs *et al.*, 2016)
85 (van den Beuken-van Everdingen *et al.*, 2007)
86 (Sennfält *et al.*, 2004)
87 (Bader *et al.*, 2012)
88 (Silva *et al.*, 2022)
89 (Walsh *et al.*, 2022)
90 (Levren *et al.*, 2011)
91 (Schaake *et al.*, 2018)
92 (Fernandes *et al.*, 2018)

about one week.[93] TAPS has been associated with decreased quality of life, influencing chemotherapy treatment doses and timing and leading to treatment discontinuation.

Cancer pain classification

According to Kumar,[94] cancer pain can be categorized into three levels of classification: symptom based, syndrome based, and mechanism based.

Symptom based classification

These can be classified as continuous or intermittent pain; and mild (1–4), moderate (5–6), and severe (7–10), on a numeric pain scale ranging from 0–10.

Syndrome based classification

These can be classified by origin, for example, from nociceptors in bone, soft tissue, or visceral structure; or by region, such as lower back, abdominal region, thoracic region, lower limbs, head, or pelvic organs.

Mechanism based classification

There are five mechanisms in pain perception, according to Kumar and Saha's mechanism based classification:[95]

- *Central sensitization* is pain mediated from higher brain centers with an absence of peripheral nociceptive stimulus. Central sensitization can occur with the presence of allodynia (pain perception in response to a non-painful stimulus) or hyperalgesia (an exaggerated response to a painful stimulus). Central pain mechanisms can be illustrated by functional anatomical changes in the somatosensory cortex, for example in the case of phantom limb pain, or by pain due to emotional phenomena occurring in cancer patients.[96] Central sensitization pain may also be triggered by a variety of stimuli, such as bright light, food, weather changes, odours, noise, and stress.[97]
- *Peripheral sensitization* is an increase in magnitude of a response (or increased sensitization) from peripheral sensory nerve fibers.[98] Peripheral sensitization can be accompanied with numbness and muscle weakness. Cancer-related peripheral sensitization causes may be attributed to chemotherapy induced neuropathy, post-radiation

93   (Loprinzi *et al.*, 2011)
94   (Kumar, 2011)
95   (Kumar & Saha, 2011)
96   (Kumar, 2011)
97   (Nijs *et al.*, 2016)
98   (Gangadharan & Kuner, 2013)

plexopathies, or surgical neuropathies.[99] This type of pain may follow a neuro-anatomical pain pattern.

- *Peripheral nociceptive* pain is a response to noxious chemical, mechanical, or thermal stimuli detected by peripheral nerve endings, or defined by activation of nociceptors due to a threat or damage to a non-neural tissue.[100] This type of pain in cancer patients may be attributed partially to musculoskeletal/fascia changes occurring from tissue disuse, deconditioning, or postural adaptations due to clinical manifestations of the disease or treatments. Musculoskeletal nociceptive pain in cancer patients, according to Kumar, is pain provoked by specific postures or movements, experienced in relevant anatomical areas, intermittent in nature, and mostly mild to moderate in nature.[101] Nociceptive pain usually relates to an injury, a pathology, or an objective dysfunction.[102]

- *Sympathetically dependent* pain can be observed in cancer patients. Evidence of "burning" and "throbbing" pain presented with allodynia, hyperpathia (delayed pain response to touch stimuli), and hypoalgesia to pin prick testing in painful sites can be signs of sympathetically dependent pain. Usually, this type of pain can be relieved by sympathetic block and will often show signs of excessive sweating and vasoconstriction.[103]

- *Cognitive-affective and psychosocial* pain is that is affected by cognitive, emotional, or social factors. Mental health conditions such as depression and anxiety can highly influence the perception of pain,[104] as well as affecting cognition, and cognitive status will also influence pain reporting characteristics. Cognitive-affective pain in cancer patients can be the result of the cancer itself, the effect of treatment, or the effect of pain medication such as opioids or narcotics.[105] Psychological characteristics such as guilt, preoccupation with pain, emotions, low ego strength, high neuroticism, low self-confidence, and high dependence on external locus of control, along with social factors such as general stressors, family and work strain, social networks, family support, social functioning, coping response, and family modelling, were associated with higher reported pain levels in cancer patients.[106]

In summary, pain is a complex phenomenon that can be influenced and caused by many factors during prostate cancer survivors' disease course.

---

99   (Paice, 2003)
100 (Nijs *et al.*, 2016)
101 (Kumar, 2011)
102 (Nijs *et al.*, 2016)
103 (Kumar, 2011)
104 (Bushnell *et al.*, 2013)
105 (Kumar, 2011)
106 (Dalton & Feuerstein, 1988)

Although pain is not a side-effect from a specific treatment, it is a very relevant topic in prostate cancer care and survivorship. Understanding pain mechanisms and classifications may help clinicians to better address prostate cancer pain.

REFERENCES

Ablove, T. (2010). Post void dribbling: Incidence and risk factors. *Neurourology and Urodynamics, 29*(3), 432–436. https://doi.org/10.1002/nau.20775

Abrams, P., Cardozo, L., Fall, M., Griffiths, D., *et al.* (2002). The standardisation of terminology of lower urinary tract function: Report from the standardisation sub-committee of the International Continence Society. *Neurourology and Urodynamics, 21*(2), 167–178. https://doi.org/10.1002/nau.10052

Abrams, P., Cardozo, L., Fall, M., Griffiths, D., *et al.* (2003). The standardisation of terminology in lower urinary tract function: Report from the standardisation sub-committee of the International Continence Society. *Urology, 61*(1), 37–49. https://doi.org/10.1016/S0090-4295(02)02243-4

Bader, P., Echtle, D., Fonteyne, V., Livadas, K., *et al.* (2012). Prostate cancer pain management: EAU guidelines on pain management. *World Journal of Urology, 30*(5), 677–686. https://doi.org/10.1007/s00345-012-0825-1

Baztan, J.J. (2005). New-onset urinary incontinence and rehabilitation outcomes in frail older patients. *Age and Ageing, 34*(2), 172–175. https://doi.org/10.1093/ageing/afi001

Burnett, A.L., Aus, G., Canby-Hagino, E.D., Cookson, M.S., *et al.* (2007). Erectile function outcome reporting after clinically localized prostate cancer treatment. *Journal of Urology, 178*(2), 597–601. https://doi.org/10.1016/j.juro.2007.03.140

Bushnell, M.C., Čeko, M., & Low, L.A. (2013). Cognitive and emotional control of pain and its disruption in chronic pain. *Nature Reviews Neuroscience, 14*(7), 502–511. https://doi.org/10.1038/nrn3516

Cash, J.C., & Glass, C.A. (2016). *Adult-Gerontology Practice Guidelines.* Springer Publishing Company. https://connect.springerpub.com/content/reference-book/978-0-8261-5931-1

Chassagne, D., Sismondi, P., Horiot, J.C., Sinistrero, G., *et al.* (1993). A glossary for reporting complications of treatment in gynecological cancers. *Radiotherapy and Oncology, 26*(3), 195–202. https://doi.org/10.1016/0167-8140(93)90260-F

Choi, J.M., Nelson, C.J., Stasi, J., & Mulhall, J.P. (2007). Orgasm associated incontinence (climacturia) following radical pelvic surgery: Rates of occurrence and predictors. *Journal of Urology, 177*(6), 2223–2226. https://doi.org/10.1016/j.juro.2007.01.150

Dalton, J.A., & Feuerstein, M. (1988). Biobehavioral factors in cancer pain. *Pain, 33*(2), 137–147. https://doi.org/10.1016/0304-3959(88)90084-X

D'Ancona, C., Haylen, B., Oelke, M., Abranches-Monteiro, L., *et al.* (2019). The International Continence Society (ICS) report on the terminology for adult male lower urinary tract and pelvic floor symptoms and dysfunction. *Neurourology and Urodynamics, 38*(2), 433–477. https://doi.org/10.1002/nau.23897

Das, A.K., Kucherov, V., Glick, L., & Chung, P. (2020). Male urinary incontinence after prostate disease treatment. *Canadian Journal of Urology, 27*(S3), 36–43.

Denham, J.W., & Hauer-Jensen, M. (2002). The radiotherapeutic injury—A complex 'wound.' *Radiotherapy and Oncology, 63*(2), 129–145. https://doi.org/10.1016/S0167-8140(02)00060-9

Denton, A.S., Clarke, N., & Maher, J. (2002). Non-surgical interventions for late radiation cystitis in patients who have received radical radiotherapy to the pelvis. *Cochrane Database of Systematic Reviews, 3.* https://doi.org/10.1002/14651858.CD001773

Edmunds, K., Tuffaha, H., Galvão, D.A., Scuffham, P., & Newton, R.U. (2020). Incidence of the adverse effects of androgen deprivation therapy for prostate cancer: A systematic literature review. *Supportive Care in Cancer, 28*(5), 2079–2093. https://doi.org/10.1007/s00520-019-05255-5

Ewertz, M., Qvortrup, C., & Eckhoff, L. (2015). Chemotherapy-induced peripheral neuropathy in patients treated with taxanes and platinum derivatives. *Acta Oncologica*, *54*(5), 587–591. https://doi.org/10.3109/0284186X.2014.995775

Felde, G., Ebbesen, M.H., & Hunskaar, S. (2017). Anxiety and depression associated with urinary incontinence. A 10-year follow-up study from the Norwegian HUNT study (EPINCONT). *Neurourology and Urodynamics*, *36*(2), 322–328. https://doi.org/10.1002/nau.22921

Fernandes, R., Ibrahim, M.F.K., Stober, C., da Costa, M., *et al.* (2018). Taxane acute pain syndrome (TAPS) in patients receiving chemotherapy for breast or prostate cancer: A prospective multi-center study. *Supportive Care in Cancer*, *26*(9), 3073–3081. https://doi.org/10.1007/s00520-018-4161-x

Ficarra, V., Novara, G., Rosen, R.C., Artibani, W., *et al.* (2012). Systematic review and meta-analysis of studies reporting urinary continence recovery after robot-assisted radical prostatectomy. *European Urology*, *62*(3), 405–417. https://doi.org/10.1016/j.eururo.2012.05.045

Gangadharan, V., & Kuner, R. (2013). Pain hypersensitivity mechanisms at a glance. *Disease Models & Mechanisms*, *6*(4), 889–895. https://doi.org/10.1242/dmm.011502

Groutz, A., Blaivas, J.G., Chaikin, D.C., Weiss, J.P., & Verhaaren, M. (2000). The pathophysiology of post-radical prostatectomy incontinence: A clinical and video urodynamic study. *Journal of Urology*, *163*(6), 1767–1770.

Gutstein, H.B. (2001). The biologic basis of fatigue. *Cancer*, *92*(S6), 1678–1683. https://acsjournals.onlinelibrary.wiley.com/toc/10970142/2001/92/S6

Helissey, C., Cavallero, S., Brossard, C., Dusaud, M., Chargari, C., & François, S. (2020). Chronic inflammation and radiation-induced cystitis: Molecular background and therapeutic perspectives. *Cells*, *10*(1), 21. https://doi.org/10.3390/cells10010021

Hoyland, K., Vasdev, N., Abrof, A., & Boustead, G. (2014). Post-radical prostatectomy incontinence: Etiology and prevention. *Reviews in Urology*, *16*(4), 181–188.

ICS2022 (n.d.). *Round Table Discussion 6—Masterclass in Post-Prostatectomy Incontinence*. ICS. Retrieved April 15, 2023 from www.ics.org/2022/session/7456.

International Association for the Study of Pain (n.d.). Terminology. Retrieved February 13, 2023 from www.iasp-pain.org/resources/terminology

Johns Hopkins Medicine (2019). Chemotherapy for prostate cancer. Retrieved on September 25, 2023, from www.hopkinsmedicine.org/health/conditions-and-diseases/prostate-cancer/chemotherapy-for-prostate-cancer

Jones, C.U., Chetner, M.P., & Rotman, M. (2011). Radiotherapy and short-term androgen deprivation for localized prostate cancer. *New England Journal of Medicine*, *12*.

Kannady, C., & Clavell Hernandez, J. (2020). Orgasm-associated urinary incontinence (climacturia) following radical prostatectomy: A review of pathophysiology and current treatment options. *Asian Journal of Andrology*, *22*. https://doi.org/10.4103/aja.aja_145_19

Katz, G., & Rodriguez, R. (2007). Changes in continence and health-related quality of life after curative treatment and watchful waiting of prostate cancer. *Urology*, *69*(6), 1157–1160. https://doi.org/10.1016/j.urology.2007.02.003

Khan, A., Crump, R.T., Carlson, K.V., & Baverstock, R.J. (2021). The relationship between overactive bladder and prostate cancer: A scoping review. *Canadian Urological Association Journal [Journal De l'Association Des Urologues Du Canada]*, *15*(9), E501–E509. https://doi.org/10.5489/cuaj.7058

Kielb, S.J., & Clemens, J.Q. (2005). Comprehensive urodynamics evaluation of 146 men with incontinence after radical prostatectomy. *Urology*, *66*(2), 392–396. https://doi.org/10.1016/j.urology.2005.03.026

Kocjancic, E., Chung, E., Garzon, J. A., Haylen, B., *et al.* (2022). International Continence Society (ICS) report on the terminology for sexual health in men with lower urinary tract (LUT) and pelvic floor (PF) dysfunction. *Neurourology and Urodynamics*, *41*(1), 140–165. https://doi.org/10.1002/nau.24846

Koguchi, T., Haga, N., Matsuoka, K., Yabe, M., *et al.* (2019). Atherosclerosis as a predictor of transient exacerbation of overactive bladder symptoms after robot-assisted laparoscopic radical prostatectomy. *International Journal of Urology: Official Journal of the Japanese Urological Association*, *26*(2), 234–240. https://doi.org/10.1111/iju.13848

Kolb, N.A., Smith, A.G., Singleton, J.R., Beck, S.L., Stoddard, G.J., Brown, S., & Mooney, K. (2016). The association of chemotherapy-induced peripheral neuropathy symptoms and the risk of falling. *JAMA Neurology*, *73*(7), 860–866. https://doi.org/10.1001/jamaneurol.2016.0383

Kumar, S.P. (2011). Cancer pain: A critical review of mechanism-based classification and physical therapy management in palliative care. *Indian Journal of Palliative Care*, *17*(2), 116–126. https://doi.org/10.4103/0973-1075.84532

Kumar, S.P., & Saha, S. (2011). Mechanism-based classification of pain for physical therapy management in palliative care: A clinical commentary. *Indian Journal of Palliative Care*, *17*(1), 80–86. https://doi.org/10.4103/0973-1075.78458

Kwong, P.W., Cumming, R.G., Chan, L., Seibel, M.J., et al. (2010). Urinary incontinence and quality of life among older community-dwelling Australian men: The CHAMP study. *Age and Ageing*, *39*(3), 349–354. https://doi.org/10.1093/ageing/afq025

Lai, H.H., Rawal, A., Shen, B., & Vetter, J. (2016). The relationship between anxiety and overactive bladder or urinary incontinence symptoms in the clinical population. *Urology*, *98*, 50–57. https://doi.org/10.1016/j.urology.2016.07.013

Leach, G.E., Trockman, B., Wong, A., Hamilton, J., Haab, F., & Zimmern, P.E. (1996). Post-prostatectomy incontinence: Urodynamic findings and treatment outcomes. *Journal of Urology*, *155*(4), 1256–1259. https://doi.org/10.1016/S0022-5347(01)66235-9

Lee, D.S., & Lee, S. (2021). Urodynamic evaluation of patients with localized prostate cancer before and 4 months after robotic radical prostatectomy. *Scientific Reports*, *11*(1), 1–8. https://doi.org/10.1038/s41598-021-83143-x

Levren, G., Sadik, M., Gjertsson, P., Lomsky, M., Michanek, A., & Edenbrandt, L. (2011). Relation between pain and skeletal metastasis in patients with prostate or breast cancer. *Clinical Physiology and Functional Imaging*, *31*(3), 193–195. https://doi.org/10.1111/j.1475-097X.2010.00999.x

Liu, M., Pickles, T., Berthelet, E., Agranovich, A., et al. (2005). Urinary incontinence in prostate cancer patients treated with external beam radiotherapy. *Radiotherapy and Oncology*, *74*(2), 197–201. https://doi.org/10.1016/j.radonc.2004.09.016

Loprinzi, C.L., Reeves, B.N., Dakhil, S.R., Sloan, J.A., et al. (2011). Natural history of paclitaxel-associated acute pain syndrome: Prospective cohort study NCCTG N08C1. *Journal of Clinical Oncology*, *29*(11), 1472–1478. https://doi.org/10.1200/JCO.2010.33.0308

Maeda, Y., Høyer, M., Lundby, L., & Norton, C. (2011). Faecal incontinence following radiotherapy for prostate cancer: A systematic review. *Radiotherapy and Oncology*, *98*(2), 145–153. https://doi.org/10.1016/j.radonc.2010.12.004

Magheli, A., & Burnett, A.L. (2009). Erectile dysfunction following prostatectomy: Prevention and treatment. *Nature Reviews Urology*, *6*(8), Article 8. https://doi.org/10.1038/nrurol.2009.126

Martin, S.E., Begun, E.M., Samir, E., Azaiza, M.T., Allegro, S., & Abdelhady, M. (2019). Incidence and morbidity of radiation-induced hemorrhagic cystitis in prostate cancer. *Urology*, *131*, 190–195. https://doi.org/10.1016/j.urology.2019.05.034

McConkey, R.W. (2016). The psychosocial dimensions of fatigue in men treated for prostate cancer. *International Journal of Urological Nursing*, *10*(1), 37–43. https://doi.org/10.1111/ijun.12089

Melotti, I.G.R., Juliato, C.R.T., Tanaka, M., & Riccetto, C.L.Z. (2018). Severe depression and anxiety in women with overactive bladder. *Neurourology and Urodynamics*, *37*(1), 223–228. https://doi.org/10.1002/nau.23277

Mock, V. (2000). NCCN practice guidelines for cancer-related fatigue: Version 2000. *Oncology (08909091)*, *14*(11A), 151–161.

Mols, F., van de Poll-Franse, L.V., Vreugdenhil, G., Beijers, A.J., Kieffer, J.M., Aaronson, N.K., & Husson, O. (2016). Reference data of the European Organisation for Research and Treatment of Cancer (EORTC) QLQ-CIPN20 Questionnaire in the general Dutch population. *European Journal of Cancer*, *69*, 28–38. https://doi.org/10.1016/j.ejca.2016.09.020

Mornex, F., Pavy, J. J., Denekamp, J., & Bolla, M. (1997). Système d'évaluation des effets tardifs des radiations sur les tissus normaux: L'échelle SOMA-LENT. *Cancer/Radiothérapie*, *1*(6), 622–627. https://doi.org/10.1016/S1278-3218(97)82941-1

Mulhall, J.P., Luo, X., Zou, K.H., Stecher, V., & Galaznik, A. (2016). Relationship between age and erectile dysfunction diagnosis or treatment using real-world observational data in the USA. *International Journal of Clinical Practice*, *70*(12), 1012–1018. https://doi.org/10.1111/ijcp.12908

Muñoz-Yagüe, T., Solís-Muñoz, P., Ciriza de los Ríos, C., Muñoz-Garrido, F., Vara, J., & Solís-Herruzo, J.A. (2014). Fecal incontinence in men: Causes and clinical and manometric features. *World Journal of Gastroenterology*, *20*(24), 7933–7940. https://doi.org/10.3748/wjg.v20.i24.7933

Murphy, D.G., Pascoe, C., Lawrentschuk, N., Davis, N.F., Duncan, C., Lamb, B.W., & Lynch, T.H. (2019). Current management of radiation cystitis: A review and practical guide to clinical management. *BJU International*, *123*(4), 585–594. https://doi.org/10.1111/bju.14516

Nickel, J.C., & Speakman, M. (2019). Post-void dribbling—Is it time to take another look at a common urology problem? *Journal of Urology*, *201*(6), 1064–1066. https://doi.org/10.1097/JU.0000000000000074

Nijs, J., Leysen, L., Adriaenssens, N., Aguilar Ferrándiz, M.E., et al. (2016). Pain following cancer treatment: Guidelines for the clinical classification of predominant neuropathic, nociceptive and central sensitization pain. *Acta Oncologica*, *55*(6), 659–663. https://doi.org/10.3109/0284186X.2016.1167958

Nilsson, A.E., Schumacher, M.C., Johansson, E., Carlsson, S., et al. (2011). Age at surgery, educational level and long-term urinary incontinence after radical prostatectomy. *BJU International*, *108*(10), 1572–1577. https://doi.org/10.1111/j.1464-410X.2011.10231.x

O'Neil, B.B., Presson, A., Gannon, J., Stephenson, R.A., et al. (2014). Climacturia after definitive treatment of prostate cancer. *Journal of Urology*, *191*(1), 159–163. https://doi.org/10.1016/j.juro.2013.06.122

Ouizeman, D.J., Marine-Barjoan, E., Hastier-De Chelles, A., De Matharel, M., Montoya, M.-L., Anty, R., & Piche, T. (2020). The severity of symptoms is insufficient to predict major alterations to quality of life of patients with fecal incontinence or chronic constipation. *International Journal of Colorectal Disease*, *35*(11), 2041–2048. https://doi.org/10.1007/s00384-020-03685-w

Paice, J.A. (2003). Mechanisms and management of neuropathic pain in cancer. *Journal of Supportive Oncology*, *1*(2), 107–120.

Pastore, A.L., Palleschi, G., Illiano, E., Zucchi, A., Carbone, A., & Costantini, E. (2017). The role of detrusor overactivity in urinary incontinence after radical prostatectomy: A systematic review. *Minerva Urologica e Nefrologica (Italian Journal of Urology and Nephrology)*, (3), 234–241. https://doi.org/10.23736/s0393-2249.16.02790-9

Rao, S.S.C. (2004). Diagnosis and management of fecal incontinence. *Official Journal of the American College of Gastroenterology* (ACG), (8), 1585–1604.

Rigaud, J., Hetet, J.-F., & Bouchot, O. (2004). [Management of radiation cystitis]. *Progres en urologie*, *14*(4), 568–572.

Salter, C.A. (2020). Perspective regarding "prevalence and predictors of climacturia and associated patient/partner bother in patients with history of definitive therapy for prostate cancer." *Journal of Sexual Medicine*, *17*(6), 1207. https://doi.org/10.1016/j.jsxm.2020.02.028

Sanguedolce, F., Sancho Pardo, G., Mercadé Sanchez, A., Balaña Lucena, J., et al. (2021). Radiation-induced haemorrhagic cystitis after prostate cancer radiotherapy: Factors associated to hospitalization and treatment strategies. *Prostate International*, *9*(1), 48–53. https://doi.org/10.1016/j.prnil.2020.07.006

Schaake, W., van der Schaaf, A., van Dijk, L.V., van den Bergh, A.C.M., & Langendijk, J.A. (2018). Development of a prediction model for late urinary incontinence, hematuria, pain and voiding frequency among irradiated prostate cancer patients. *PloS One*, *13*(7), e0197757. https://doi.org/10.1371/journal.pone.0197757

Sennfält, K., Carlsson, P., Sandblom, G., & Varenhorst, E. (2004). The estimated economic value of the welfare loss due to prostate cancer pain in a defined population. *Acta Oncologica (Stockholm, Sweden)*, *43*(3), 290–296. https://doi.org/10.1080/02841860410028411

Seretny, M., Currie, G.L., Sena, E.S., Ramnarine, S., et al. (2014). Incidence, prevalence, and predictors of chemotherapy-induced peripheral neuropathy: A systematic review and meta-analysis. *PAIN®*, *155*(12), 2461–2470. https://doi.org/10.1016/j.pain.2014.09.020

Silva, T.B., Cardoso, M.A.S., Ramim, J.E., Bergmann, A., & Pujatti, P.B. (2022). Single-center, retrospective study on changes in pain-relieving therapy after bone metastasis detection by bone scintigraphy in prostate cancer patients. *Brazilian Journal of Pharmaceutical Sciences, 58*. https://doi.org/10.1590/s2175-97902022e191058

Stasi, R., Abriani, L., Beccaglia, P., Terzoli, E., & Amadori, S. (2003). Cancer-related fatigue. *Cancer, 98*(9), 1786–1801. https://doi.org/10.1002/cncr.11742

Tal, R., Alphs, H.H., Krebs, P., Nelson, C.J., & Mulhall, J.P. (2009). Erectile function recovery rate after radical prostatectomy: A meta-analysis. *Journal of Sexual Medicine, 6*(9), 2538–2546. https://doi.org/10.1111/j.1743-6109.2009.01351.x

Tatenuma, T., Makiyama, K., Ito, Y., Muraoka, K., et al. (2021). Correlation of urinary loss rate after catheter removal and long-term urinary continence after robot-assisted laparoscopic radical prostatectomy. *International Journal of Urology, 28*(4), 440–443. https://doi.org/10.1111/iju.14488

Tienza, A., Robles, J.E., Hevia, M., Algarra, R., Diez-Caballero, F., & Pascual, J.I. (2018). Prevalence analysis of urinary incontinence after radical prostatectomy and influential preoperative factors in a single institution. *The Aging Male, 21*(1), 24–30. https://doi.org/10.1080/13685538.2017.1369944

Twitchell, D.K., Wittmann, D.A., Hotaling, J.M., & Pastuszak, A.W. (2019). Psychological impacts of male sexual dysfunction in pelvic cancer survivorship. *Sexual Medicine Reviews, 7*(4), 614–626. https://doi.org/10.1016/j.sxmr.2019.02.003

van den Beuken-van Everdingen, M.H.J., de Rijke, J.M., Kessels, A.G., Schouten, H.C., van Kleef, M., & Patijn, J. (2007). High prevalence of pain in patients with cancer in a large population-based study in The Netherlands. *Pain, 132*(3), 312–320. https://doi.org/10.1016/j.pain.2007.08.022

Walsh, E.A., Pedreira, P.B., Moreno, P.I., Popok, P.J., et al. (2022). Pain, cancer-related distress, and physical and functional well-being among men with advanced prostate cancer. *Supportive Care in Cancer, 31*(1), 28–28. https://doi.org/10.1007/s00520-022-07453-0

Wei, J.T., & Montie, J.E. (2000). Comparison of patients' and physicians' rating of urinary incontinence following radical prostatectomy. *Seminars in Urologic Oncology, 18*(1), 76–80.

Wilson, L.C., & Gilling, P.J. (2011). Post-prostatectomy urinary incontinence: A review of surgical treatment options. *BJU International, 107*, 7–10. https://doi.org/10.1111/j.1464-410X.2011.10052.x

Yalla, S.V., Dibenedetto, M., Fam, B.A., Blunt, K.J., Constantinople, N., & Gabilondo, F.B. (1979). Striated sphincter participation in distal passive urinary continence mechanisms: Studies in male subjects deprived of proximal sphincter mechanism. *Journal of Urology, 122*(5), 655–660. https://doi.org/10.1016/s0022-5347(17)56546-5

Yalla, S.V., Karsh, L., Kearney, G., Fraser, L., Finn, D., DeFelippo, N., & Dyro, F.M. (1982). Postprostatectomy urinary incontinence: Urodynamic assessment. *Neurourology and Urodynamics, 1*(1), 77–87. https://doi.org/10.1002/nau.1930010107

Zajączkowska, R., Kocot-Kępska, M., Leppert, W., Wrzosek, A., Mika, J., & Wordliczek, J. (2019). Mechanisms of chemotherapy-induced peripheral neuropathy. *International Journal of Molecular Sciences, 20*(6), Article 6. https://doi.org/10.3390/ijms20061451

Zwaans, B.M.M., Wegner, K.A., Bartolone, S.N., Vezina, C.M., Chancellor, M.B., & Lamb, L.E. (2020). Radiation cystitis modeling: A comparative study of bladder fibrosis radio-sensitivity in C57BL/6, C3H, and BALB/c mice. *Physiological Reports, 8*(4), e14377. https://doi.org/10.14814/phy2.14377

PART 2

THE BIOPSYCHOSOCIAL APPROACH IN CARING FOR PROSTATE CANCER SURVIVORS

CHAPTER 5

The Biopsychosocial Model in Prostate Cancer Care

Biopsychosocial (BPS) health is based on shifting from a biomedical, organ-oriented model of care to a more integrated approach that recognizes the interconnectedness of biological, psychological, and social factors in health and illness. This approach fosters human connections in a compassionate, patient-centered, and culturally safe environment.

This chapter will introduce the characteristics of the biopsychosocial model as proposed by George Engel, including some of its modern interpretations and research data on BPS in cancer survivorship. It will also describe a few examples of training models for the integration of BPS and compassionate care in healthcare practices. Lastly, it will present the meaning of cultural safety care and how it may be integrated within a BPS model.

INTRODUCTION TO THE BIOPSYCHOSOCIAL MODEL

The biopsychosocial healthcare model, proposed by George Engel in 1977,[1] has been studied, reviewed, interpreted, and slowly applied to healthcare, including physiotherapy practices. This model of care was presented due to Engel's dissatisfaction with the current biomedical model, which in his opinion was separatist and non-integrative. He believed that complex health concerns were only addressed via biochemical or pathoanatomical processes, leaving no room for "the social, psychological, and behavioral dimensions of illness"[2]. Since then, this care model has been implemented into various healthcare settings, especially by facilities or professionals treating chronic illnesses. Its true interpretation has been questioned, as some frameworks do not utilize the humanistic approach of the biopsychosocial model[3]. For example, some models mostly focus on *causation* or solely determining the

---

1   (Engel, 1977)
2   (Engel, 1977)
3   (Cormack *et al.*, 2022)

root of the disease and dysfunction, while overlooking the importance of an ongoing *human relationship* between the client and healthcare professionals.[4]

The basis of the biopsychosocial model intends to consider all elements that can influence human beings in relation to their health and their ability to respond to recovering from illnesses and conditions. This principle can be achieved by integrating biological, psychological, and social factors for every healthcare task.[5, 6] More specifically, it theoretically fosters the importance of *person-centered care, therapeutic alliance, self-management* approach and individualized *meaningful goal setting*.[7]

Person-centered care

Person-centered care puts patients (their families, caregivers, or representatives) at the forefront of their healthcare journey. The people searching for health benefits—including prevention or promotion of activities—or patients wanting to improve a condition or an illness, are seen as individuals who are unique, and have different perspectives, goals, concerns, and needs.[8] Patients and healthcare professionals are encouraged to co-design their treatment plans to provide individualized care, where goals are set in a meaningful way for those individuals seeking care.[9] Person-centered care is achieved by *active listening* through verbal and non-verbal communication, providing information for *informed decision making* related to their diagnosis and treatment plan, and acknowledging their social and cultural values, and that they are also an expert of their own health journey.[10]

Therapeutic alliance

Therapeutic alliance highlights the importance to foster and strengthen clinician–patient relationship on the basis that this strong relationship can highly influence therapeutic outcome. *Empathy* and *establishing meaningful connections* seem to be key elements that can contribute to a strong therapeutic alliance.[11, 12] Empathy is the ability to bring awareness of others' feelings and emotions, and to be able to place oneself in another's position.[13] Empathy in healthcare translates into developing a cognitive behavior that allows clinicians to understand the unique perspective and experiences of "patients", and being able to communicate that understanding back to them. There is

---

4   (Cormack *et al.*, 2022)
5   (Smith *et al.*, 2013)
6   (Molyneux, 2022)
7   (Cormack *et al.*, 2022)
8   (Santana *et al.*, 2018)
9   (Santana *et al.*, 2018)
10 (Santana *et al.*, 2018)
11 (Hutting *et al.*, 2022)
12 (Paul-Savoie *et al.*, 2018)
13 (Bellet & Maloney, 1991)

evidence to support that a clinician's empathy can help to reduce distress, enhance compliance, and improve the patient's satisfaction. More specifically, it can reduce depression and improve the quality of life of cancer patients receiving care.[14, 15] An empathetic communication can facilitate healthcare practitioners to receive more information related to symptoms, concerns, and psychosocial situations of the individuals seeking care, which in turn can help clinicians develop a more effective treatment plan.[16]

Fostering a strong therapeutic alliance can strengthen a trusting connection and mutual understanding between patient and clinician, and can promote positive health education; it is probably the central component to a humanistic biopsychosocial model.[17]

Self-management

Many programs geared towards individuals with chronic conditions and persistent pain have utilized self-management approaches to empower these individuals with knowledge and tools in the aim to make them active participants of their health path and optimal function.[18] Self-management fosters strong communication skills between the individual and healthcare practitioners with the goal of increasing the individual's role into managing their health. These elements of person-centered and meaningful communication strategies align well with the biopsychosocial framework. These were important skills reported to be learned during self-management programs:[19]

- Goal setting
- Shared decision making
- Problem solving
- Action planning
- Forming partnerships.

Enactivism and the modern interpretations of the biopsychosocial model[20]

Enactivist theories combine the humanistic and causation biopsychosocial approach proposed by Engel, with the additional focus of the individuals' perceived relationship and interaction with their social and physical environment. These theorists suggest that people's experiences, such as pain or dysfunction, can be influenced by how they may envision their interactions with the world they live in. For example, people living with chronic conditions

---

14 (Neumann *et al.*, 2007)
15 (Thomas *et al.*, 2021)
16 (Neumann *et al.*, 2007)
17 (Cormack *et al.*, 2022)
18 (Barlow *et al.*, 2002)
19 (Hutting *et al.*, 2022)
20 (Cormack *et al.*, 2022)

may picture their world as more threatening, or believe themselves as not whole, restricting the interaction with their environment. This consequently may foster maladaptive behaviors such as fear, avoidance, isolation, and sense of hopelessness, and limit their participation into meaningful activities. Enactivism theorists, such as Stilwell and Harman, conceptualized the idea that symptoms experienced are not only related to bodily tissues, or the brain, but are also influenced by a sense-making body that is *relational and emergent* and is "inseparable from the world that we shape and that shapes us."[21]

Compassion in healthcare

Goetz and colleagues describe compassion as a form of awareness to pain and suffering with the *desire and motivation* to alleviate the pain and suffering (of self and of others).[22] Compassion may differ from empathy, as empathic behavior is not usually associated with the desire to relieve one's suffering. Empathy, different from compassion, can sometimes lead to negative affect, for example experiencing negative emotions in response to someone in distress.[23]

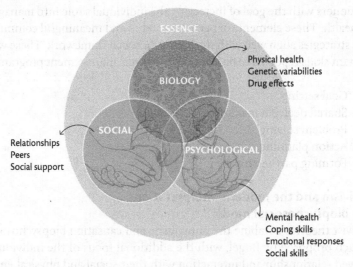

ESSENCE

BIOLOGY

Physical health
Genetic variabilities
Drug effects

SOCIAL

Relationships
Peers
Social support

PSYCHOLOGICAL

Mental health
Coping skills
Emotional responses
Social skills

FIGURE 5.1: THE BIOPSYCHOSOCIAL MODEL IN CANCER CARE

Introducing compassion into biopsychosocial models of care may deepen the connection between individuals and healthcare professionals and strengthen therapeutic alliance. It was suggested that compassionate care has positive effects on health such as improving mental and physical wellbeing and

---

21   (Stilwell & Harman, 2019)
22   (Goetz *et al.*, 2017)
23   (Seppälä *et al.*, 2017)

reducing stress and anxiety.[24] Arman and Hok's study demonstrated that compassionate care from health professionals may be the driving force for women with persistent pain to follow through with active self-management and care.[25] Moreover, Halifax suggests that compassion is particularly relevant for healthcare providers who work with individuals with catastrophic diseases or illnesses,[26] supporting the use of compassion towards the cancer population.

CANCER SURVIVORSHIP AND THE BIOPSYCHOSOCIAL MODEL

Prostate cancer can be a traumatic life-altering disease with significant psychosocial impacts, affecting a multitude of life domains.[27] The American Cancer Society and other health organizations highlight the importance of prostate cancer survivorship programs, which include not only surveillance for prostate cancer recurrence and screening for secondary or primary cancers, but also management of long-term physical side-effects, psychosocial management, and care coordination.[28, 29, 30]

Physiotherapists and oncology professionals adopting a biopsychosocial model in prostate cancer care may facilitate the integration of all interconnecting pieces responsible for improving patients' symptoms and quality of life, as psychological wellness, social integration, and supportive and compassionate care have been linked to improving prostate cancer symptoms and survivorship.[31, 32] It may also help clinicians to view prostate cancer as a disease that challenges society's customs, rituals, and behaviors, rather than uniquely "a problem of cellular pathology rooted in biology," changing the focus of curing a disease (pathogenesis) to promoting health and healing (salutogenesis).[33]

Humanistic biopsychosocial or holistic healthcare models may improve cancer patients' outcomes. As an example, a humanistic nursing care model post ovarian cancer surgery reduced patients' hospital stay, accelerated first time ambulation, reduced self-scored anxiety and depression, and improved cortisol and blood sugar levels compared to "routine nursing intervention." This study also showed an improved level of nursing satisfaction with care

---

24 (Prosko, 2019)
25 (Arman & Hok, 2016)
26 (Halifax, 2012)
27 (Sylvestro *et al.*, 2021)
28 (Skolarus *et al.*, 2014)
29 (Howell *et al.*, 2011)
30 (Crawford-Williams *et al.*, 2018)
31 (Costanzo *et al.*, 2011)
32 (Fuertes *et al.*, 2007)
33 (Fries, 2020)

compared to control.[34] Another study demonstrated that a strong therapeutic alliance—measured by increased patient's trust, respect, and perception of doctor's concern with their quality of life—between oncologists and advanced cancer patients may be associated with better quality of life.[35] In prostate cancer care, social support and psychosocial interventions may improve stress, depression, anxiety, fatigue, and overall life satisfaction.[36, 37, 38, 39, 40]

As previously highlighted, prostate cancer survivors may continue to experience symptoms long-term or even permanently throughout their lifespan. As a result of the cancer and symptoms experienced throughout their cancer care continuum, this population is at increased risk of reduced quality of life and increased levels of anxiety and depression.[41, 42] Interventions and care using a biopsychosocial approach may help to create strong bonds and trust between therapists and prostate cancer survivors, helping to identify all the components linked to their complaints, facilitating treatment approaches, and enriching the opportunity for improving outcomes. Taking in consideration people's lives and their environment as part of healthcare screening may further improve their sense of purpose and quality of life.

CULTURAL SAFETY IN CANCER CARE

Cultural safety in cancer care is concerned with improving the stigma, prejudice, power relationship, and attitude of healthcare workers (physiotherapists, nurses, physicians) towards their patients who may differ in gender, sexuality, ethnicity, social class, cultural background, generation, or other variables.[43] The implementation of cultural safety and recognizing cultural needs of society's marginalized groups, such as Indigenous peoples, immigrants, or Black or Asian people, may influence their access to cancer care in timely manners. Marginalized people experiencing social inequities may have higher rates of advanced cancer at diagnosis and cancer mortality, perhaps due to being less likely to access care and treatment from a more regimented biomedical model of care.[44] This effect may be attributed by multiple levels of influences, including patients' and families' cultural beliefs leading to misunderstandings and fears pertaining to prostate cancer,[45] and

34   (Gao et al., 2021)
35   (Thomas et al., 2021)
36   (Jan et al., 2016)
37   (Zhao et al., 2021)
38   (Colloca & Colloca, 2016)
39   (Chien et al., 2014)
40   (McConkey, 2016)
41   (Watts et al., 2014)
42   (Massoeurs et al., 2021)
43   (Ramsden, 2002)
44   (Horrill et al., 2022)
45   (Vapiwala et al., 2021)

patients and oncology providers' biases in the decision-making process of managing the illness. These biases may occur due to beliefs, assumptions, or negative unconscious feelings toward a different group (cultural, social-economic, race, etc.), which may provoke shorter, negative, or non-effective interactions between patients and clinicians, and may consequently result in poorer cancer patients' health outcomes.[46] Power imbalances from clinicians and patients may result in decreased shared decision making during their cancer journey,[47] and can be especially detrimental to the health status of "colonized" people, such as Indigenous peoples in Australia, Canada, and the United States.[48]

Fostering trust, emotional safety, and changing power-relationships between oncology practitioners and patients may be necessary in cancer care models to improve social groups' outcomes. Culturally-sensitive education may strengthen therapeutic alliances between clinicians and patients with ethnic or cultural disparities[49] fostering compassionate patient-centered cancer care.

PRACTICAL APPLICATIONS OF THE BIOPSYCHOSOCIAL MODEL

How can healthcare professionals and physiotherapists apply some of the main concepts of the biopsychosocial model into their cancer care practices?

The complexity and different interpretations its biopsychosocial model may offer barriers to effectively applying its theories into practice. For example, one may interpret the model as strictly determining the root of the disease within its biological, psychological, and social aspects without fostering the importance of a humanistic approach. Also, clinicians' biases, past experiences, and cultural values without cultural safety and humility training may limit clinicians' integration of a client-centered compassionate care.

Behaviorally defined interviewing methods, such as *motivational interviewing* or patient-centered interviewing (proposed by Smith and colleagues[50]) and compassion fostering training, may facilitate a humanistic BPS approach in addressing prostate cancer care. Moreover, examining power dynamics in clinician–patient relationships,[51] acknowledging decision-making biases, and identifying barriers to facilitate inclusive care may improve cultural safety practices.

---

46   (Vo *et al.*, 2021)
47   (Joseph-Williams *et al.*, 2014)
48   (Durey *et al.*, 2017)
49   (Elliott-Groves, 2019)
50   (Smith *et al.*, 2013)
51   (Boyd, 1996)

Motivational interviewing

Motivational interviewing (MI) is a *communication style* that is centered in collaboration, partnership, and empathy, while emphasizing the individual's autonomy.[52] It was shaped into a more detailed clinical method of counseling by the psychologists William Miller and Stephen Rollnick for the purpose of encouraging health-related behavioral changes in ambivalent substance-abuse patients.[53] MI is a philosophy and a communication style viewing *ambivalence* with curiosity and acceptance while evoking individuals' hopes, values, and priorities. It is an open-style, empathetic, and 'curious' form of communication that will guide more than direct, listen *as much as* speak, and will seek more understanding rather than judge.[54] This collaborative approach aims to elicit individuals to verbalize their reasons for making a behavioral change and barriers they are facing, rather than being solely passive listeners.

MI has been applied in numerous healthcare settings, and has been shown to be beneficial for healthy behavioral changes, such as smoking cessation and weight loss.[55] Some of its core communication strategies include:

- Listening for change talk
- Open-ended questions
- Affirmations
- Reflections
- Summaries
- Informing and advising

Motivational interviewing's communication strategies[56]
Listening for change talk

During a conversation, listening for change talk is commenting, highlighting, or reflecting on the individuals' desire to change or the importance of change, rather than focusing on why the change isn't or can't happen. It has been shown that the patient's verbalization of change talk is predictive of future healthy behavioral change.[57]

---

52 (Rubak *et al.*, 2005)
53 (Miller & Rollnick, 2012)
54 (Treasure, 2004)
55 (Childers *et al.*, 2012)
56 Based on the book *Motivational Interviewing: Helping People Change, Third Edition* (Miller & Rollnick, 2012)
57 (Apodaca & Longabaugh, 2009)

Open-ended questions

An open-ended question is the type of question that has answers different from a simple yes or no. Open-ended questions may elicit more "change talk" and can be a simple way of enriching patient–clinician interaction. It may also result in receiving more information from the patient or individual's desire to change and their confidence in their ability to do so. For example, when trying to obtain a patient's desire to exercise, it could be asked: "What changes do you think you need in order to implement an exercise program into your routine?" or "What are the health benefits you think you'll get by exercising?" or even "Why is exercise important to you?"

Table 5.1: Examples of close- and open-ended questions

Closed-ended questions	Open-ended questions
Do you get enough sleep?	What are your sleeping habits like?
Does your back hurt?	How would you describe how your back feels?
Are you drinking enough water?	What is your fluid intake like on a regular basis?
Did you practice your exercises?	What was your exercise routine like this week?

Affirmations

Affirmations are positive acknowledgments recognizing an individual's strength and behavior leading towards positive change. It may strengthen an individual's self-efficacy or perception of his/her ability to be able to make positive changes. For example, one can say: " I can see you are taking positive steps towards building up your stamina," or " It shows that you care for your health." Affirmations can be used as a way to express that you care!

Reflections

Reflections are reinstatements of what was said by the individual or the patient. Reflection can be used to enhance connection, for clarification, and to create some space for change talk. It can also slow things down to allow the patient's emotional reflections. Reflections can state ambivalence or show the individual the two sides of a story. This can help to reinstate the reasons for change and the obstacles to change. Usually as a rule of thumb, when reinstating the barriers and reasons for change, first reflect on the barriers, leaving reflecting on the reasons for changes until last. Normally, people will remember the last thing that was said the most, and they may leave their appointments more motivated for change.

Summaries

Summaries are a way of bringing all the information together or condensing the content, in order to demonstrate accuracy in receiving the content being said. Summaries may prompt further elaboration to their wishes, concerns, ideas, and solutions. They may also evoke reflective thoughts and feelings. When summarizing, phrases such as "To sum up...", "In essence ...", and "Let me see if I understood what was said..." can be used.

Informing and advising

A clinician can still offer valuable advice within the motivational interviewing framework. The way the advice is given may differ from a more hierarchical doctor–patient approach. For example, this method of sharing information may begin by asking the person for permission for giving the advice. The information given is framed in a *sandwich* format—it is used together with communication strategies mentioned above (for example, the use of affirmations or reflections). The person or individuals receiving the information participates by sharing how much they know on the topic or are asked to see if they understood what was shared. Miller and Rollnick suggest using the method ASK-TELL-ASK when offering advice. Ask first for permission or information one already knows on the topic. Then share advice in a respectful and neutral manner and give information that *fits* the person and that is relevant to the *present*. Finally, ask for the person's thoughts or understanding.

For improving motivational interviewing skills, it may be recommended to attend a workshop, or practice with a colleague or a family member the newly learned communication strategies. *Motivational Interviewing: Helping People Change* by Miller and Rollnick also has many practical applications to enrich the learning process.[58]

FIVE-STEP PATIENT-CENTERED INTERVIEWING METHOD

A standardized patient-centered interviewing method was proposed by Smith and colleagues in 2013. This method includes the following steps:[59]

Step 1
Setting the stage for the interview by personalizing the interaction, ensuring patient comfort and privacy, and removing any barriers to communication.

---

58 (Miller & Rollnick, 2012)
59 (Smith *et al.*, 2013)

Step 2
Summarizing the patient's chief concerns and reviewing the agenda.

Step 3
Introducing the history-taking process by using attentive listening and open-ended questions.

Step 4
Discussing the physical, emotional, and social components of the patient-centered history of present illness with empathetic care.

Step 5
Summarizing the patient's story and transitioning to the doctor-centered history of present illness.

These steps are designed to ensure that the patient feels heard, understood, and involved in their care. By following this standard method, healthcare providers can gather the necessary information to provide a comprehensive and personalized treatment plan for patients, which takes into account the biopsychosocial model.

Compassion training

There is evidence that compassion may be a trainable trait (for example by practicing loving-kindness meditation[60] and yoga[61]), or can be cultivated by training non-compassion elements, which may be directly related to compassion.[62]

Halifax presented a paper on *a heuristic model of enactive compassion*, which highlights that compassion is an emergent process arising from the interaction of non-compassion elements. The author outlined six trainable *non-linear* and *co-emergent* domains that can set the field for the "emergence of compassion."[63] Table 5.2 summarizes the meaning and training suggestions of these domains.

---

60 (Seppälä *et al.*, 2014)
61 (Prosko, 2019)
62 (Halifax, 2012)
63 (Halifax, 2012)

Table 5.2: Training suggestions of the six domains of the
Heuristic Model of Enactive Compassion,
Adapted from Halifax, 2012[64] and Prosko, 2019[65]

Domain	Meaning	Clinician training
Attentional	Non-judgmental or non-reactive attention to oneself and to others	• To be fully present with mind and body sensations during patient interactions: train to keep the mind from wandering; listen to the breath and body sensations during the interaction • Mindfulness practices
Affective	The domain of cultivating positive emotions such as kindness and to maintain mental stability especially during difficult situations (equanimity)	• Practice loving-kindness meditation • Learn to increase emotional awareness • Learn to regulate emotions during patient interaction
Intentional	The ability to guide the mind of the "intention to transform suffering"	• Set intentions before patient interactions such as: "I intend to be present for the patient; I intend to pay attention to my body signs; I intend to help reduce my patient's suffering"
Insightful	The revelation or increased clarity for the people's suffering; it combines sense making without attaching the desire to a specific outcome	• Practicing "therapeutic humility" • Open to numerous outcomes that could be emergent
Embodying	Being connected with sensory and motor body input in relation to emotions experienced	• Practicing yoga • Being connected with the body sensations during interactions • Grounding technique such as feeling feet connection to the floor, or connecting with movements occurring with breathing

64 (Halifax, 2012)
65 (Prosko, 2019)

Engaged	The readiness to act upon ethical behaviors towards a compassionate response; a response from cultivating the above domains can result in engagement, such as active listening, offering consensual devices, or allowing space to patients when needed	• Practicing motivational interviewing • Self-care and self-compassion practices • Ending the patient-clinician interaction with an action representing completion, such as an exhale or handwashing with completion intentions

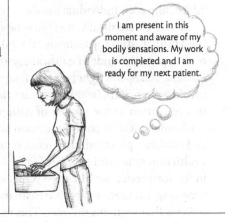

I am present in this moment and aware of my bodily sensations. My work is completed and I am ready for my next patient.

Practicing self-compassion

One may say that it may be difficult to provide compassionate care if one has low self-compassion. According to Kristin Neff, PhD, a world-renowned psychologist researcher, self-compassion is "turning compassion inwards," and can be a very powerful way to overcome life challenges while promoting mental and physical wellbeing.[66] Dr. Neff defines self-compassion as a way to offer understanding and kindness to oneself during difficult times and failures. She further elaborates that having self-compassion is embracing and honoring imperfectness. She outlines that 1. *self-kindness vs. self-judgement,* 2. *common humanity vs. isolation* and 3. *mindfulness vs. over-identification* are the three key elements for self-compassion.[67] Self-compassion practices are linked to improving therapists' empathy, and may help to facilitate compassionate care[68]. Physiotherapists and oncology workers may also use self-compassion practices as ways to improve psychological wellness and resilience. These practices will be discussed further in Chapter 9.

66 (Neff, n.d.)
67 (Neff, n.d.)
68 (Bibeau *et al.*, 2016)

Practical applications of the biopsychosocial model in healthcare may still be at its primitive stages. Currently, healthcare spending is still largely directed at biomedical interventions, neglecting social and behavioral science within clinical medicine.[69] The organ approach to medicine also places a challenge to addressing issues which may need a more integrative application. Medicine and clinicians adhering to guidelines may contribute to generalization of practice rather than addressing each individual needs.

Social-economically, there may be several obstacles to implementing a humanistic biopsychosocial model in our world healthcare system. In publicly funded healthcare systems like those found in the UK, Canada, and Spain, tight budgets, long waitlists, and limited time allocated to physicians, healthcare practitioners, and programs can result in a reduction in the quality of patient–provider interactions. This can hinder effective communication and limit the amount of support and guidance provided to patients, potentially impacting their overall health outcomes and quality of life. Prostate cancer patients residing in fee-for-service healthcare systems may face significant barriers to accessing integrative care due to financial constraints and insurance policies that segment services. This may limit their ability to receive comprehensive and holistic care, leaving them with few options for managing the physical and emotional side-effects of their treatment. Poorer countries with limited resources and decreased individual autonomy due to decreased economical and educational status may challenge the ability to implement biopsychosocial models.[70] Furthermore, the inability for individuals in low-income countries to retain and understand information about their health status (low health literacy) may make it difficult for the adoption of person-centered models and self-management programs.

CONCLUSION

This chapter offers physiotherapists and healthcare providers a different outlook to prostate cancer survivorship care. The biopsychosocial model may allow clinicians to expand their practices into treating prostate cancer survivors with a more integrative approach. Adopting a humanistic and compassionate perspective while integrating people's social and spiritual values

---

69   (Fava & Sonino, 2017)
70   (Hutting *et al.*, 2022)

may improve treatment outcomes, psychological responses, and quality of life of prostate cancer survivors.[71]

REFERENCES

Apodaca, T.R., & Longabaugh, R. (2009). Mechanisms of change in Motivational Interviewing: A review and preliminary evaluation of the evidence. *Addiction (Abingdon, England)*, *104*(5), 705–715. https://doi.org/10.1111/j.1360-0443.2009.02527.x

Arman, M., & Hok, J. (2016). Self-care follows from compassionate care – chronic pain patients' experience of integrative rehabilitation. *Scandinavian Journal of Caring Sciences 30*, 374–381.

Barlow, J., Wright, C., Sheasby, J., Turner, A., & Hainsworth, J. (2002). Self-management approaches for people with chronic conditions: A review. *Patient Education and Counseling*, *48*(2), 177–187. https://doi.org/10.1016/S0738-3991(02)00032-0

Bellet, P.S., & Maloney, M.J. (1991). The importance of empathy as an interviewing skill in medicine. *JAMA*, *266*(13), 1831–1832. https://doi.org/10.1001/jama.1991.03470130111039

Bibeau, M., Dionne, F., & Leblanc, J. (2016). Can compassion meditation contribute to the development of psychotherapists' empathy? A review. *Mindfulness*, *7*(1), 255–263. https://doi.org/10.1007/s12671-015-0439-y

Boyd, K.K. (1996). Power imbalances and therapy. *Focus: A Guide to AIDS Research and Counseling*, *11*(9).

Chien, C.-H., Liu, K.-L., Chien, H.-T., & Liu, H.-E. (2014). The effects of psychosocial strategies on anxiety and depression of patients diagnosed with prostate cancer: A systematic review. *International Journal of Nursing Studies*, *51*(1), 28–38. https://doi.org/10.1016/j.ijnurstu.2012.12.019

Childers, J.W., Bost, J.E., Kraemer, K.L., Cluss, P.A., Spagnoletti, C.L., Gonzaga, A.M.R., & Arnold, R.M. (2012). Giving residents tools to talk about behavior change: A motivational interviewing curriculum description and evaluation. *Patient Education and Counseling*, *89*(2), 281–287. https://doi.org/10.1016/j.pec.2012.08.001

Colloca, G., & Colloca, P. (2016). The effects of social support on health-related quality of life of patients with metastatic prostate cancer. *Journal of Cancer Education: Official Journal of the American Association for Cancer Education*, *31*(2), 244–252. https://doi.org/10.1007/s13187-015-0884-2

Cormack, B., Stilwell, P., Coninx, S., & Gibson, J. (2022). The biopsychosocial model is lost in translation: From misrepresentation to an enactive modernization. *Physiotherapy Theory and Practice*, *39*(11) 1–16. https://doi.org/10.1080/09593985.2022.2080130

Costanzo, E.S., Sood, A.K., & Lutgendorf, S.K. (2011). Biobehavioral influences on cancer progression. *Immunology and Allergy Clinics*, *31*(1), 109–132. https://doi.org/10.1016/j.iac.2010.09.001

Crawford-Williams, F., March, S., Goodwin, B.C., *et al.* (2018). Interventions for prostate cancer survivorship: A systematic review of reviews. *Psycho-Oncology*, *27*(10), 2339–2348. https://doi.org/10.1002/pon.4888

Durey, A., Halkett, G., Berg, M., Lester, L., & Kickett, M. (2017). Does one workshop on respecting cultural differences increase health professionals' confidence to improve the care of Australian Aboriginal patients with cancer? An evaluation. *BMC Health Services Research*, *17*(1), 660. https://doi.org/10.1186/s12913-017-2599-z

Elliott-Groves, E. (2019). A culturally-grounded biopsychosocial assessment utilizing indigenous ways of knowing with the Cowichan tribes. *Journal of Ethnic & Cultural Diversity in Social Work*, *28*(1), 115–133. https://doi.org/10.1080/15313204.2019.1570889

Engel, G.L. (1977). The need for a new medical model: A challenge for biomedicine. *Science*, *196*(4286), 129–136. https://doi.org/10.1126/science.847460

---

71 (Gao *et al.*, 2021)

Fava, G.A., & Sonino, N. (2017). From the lesson of George Engel to current knowledge: The biopsychosocial model 40 years later. *Psychotherapy and Psychosomatics, 86*(5), 257–259. https://doi.org/10.1159/000478808

Fries, C.J. (2020). The medicalization of cancer as socially constructed and culturally negotiated. *Health Promotion International, 35*(6), 1543–1550. https://doi.org/10.1093/heapro/daaa004

Fuertes, J.N., Mislowack, A., Bennett, J., Paul, L., Gilbert, T.C., Fontan, G., & Boylan, L.S. (2007). The physician–patient working alliance. *Patient Education and Counseling, 66*(1), 29–36. https://doi.org/10.1016/j.pec.2006.09.013

Gao, M., Zhang, L., Wang, Y., Li, L., Wang, C., Shen, Q., & Liao, B. (2021). Influence of humanistic care based on Carolina care model for ovarian cancer patients on postoperative recovery and quality of life. *American Journal of Translational Research, 13*(4), 3390–3399.

Goetz, J.L., & Simon-Thomas, E. (2017) The landscape of compassion: Definitions and scientific approaches. In E.M. Seppälä, E. Simon-Thomas, S.L. Brown, M.C. Worline, C.D. Cameron, & J.R. Doty (eds). *The Oxford Handbook of Compassion Science, 1st edition.* Oxford: Oxford University Press.

Halifax, J. (2012). A heuristic model of enactive compassion. *Current Opinion in Supportive and Palliative Care, 6*(2), 228–235. https://doi.org/10.1097/SPC.0b013e3283530fbe

Horrill, T.C., Browne, A.J., & Stajduhar, K.I. (2022). Equity-oriented healthcare: What it is and why we need it in oncology. *Current Oncology, 29*(18), 186–192. https://doi.org/10.3390/curroncol29010018

Howell, D., Hack, T.F., Oliver, T.K., Chulak, T., *et al.* (2011). Survivorship services for adult cancer populations: A pan-Canadian guideline. *Current Oncology, 18*(6), e265–e281.

Hutting, N., Caneiro, J.P., Ong'wen, O.M., Miciak, M., & Roberts, L. (2022). Patient-centered care in musculoskeletal practice: Key elements to support clinicians to focus on the person. *Musculoskeletal Science and Practice, 57*, 102434. https://doi.org/10.1016/j.msksp.2021.102434

Jan, M., Bonn, S.E., Sjölander, A., Wiklund, F., *et al.* (2016). The roles of stress and social support in prostate cancer mortality. *Scandinavian Journal of Urology, 50*(1), 47–55. https://doi.org/10.3109/21681805.2015.1079796

Joseph-Williams, N., Edwards, A., & Elwyn, G. (2014). Power imbalance prevents shared decision making. *BMJ, 348*(May 14, 7), g3178–g3178. https://doi.org/10.1136/bmj.g3178

Massoeurs, L., Ilie, G., Lawen, T., MacDonald, C., *et al.* (2021). Psychosocial and functional predictors of mental disorder among prostate cancer survivors: Informing survivorship care programs with evidence-based knowledge. *Current Oncology, 28*(5), 3918–3931. https://doi.org/10.3390/curroncol28050334

McConkey, R.W. (2016). The psychosocial dimensions of fatigue in men treated for prostate cancer. *International Journal of Urological Nursing, 10*(1), 37–43. https://doi.org/10.1111/ijun.12089

Miller, W.R., & Rollnick, S. (2012). *Motivational Interviewing: Helping People Change, 3rd Edition.* New York: Guilford Press.

Molyneux, C. (2022). Patient-centred care and the biopsychosocial model. *Wounds UK, 18*(1), 69–71.

Neff, K. (n.d.). Self-Compassion Exercises by Dr. Kristin Neff. Retrieved December 6, 2022 from https://self-compassion.org/category/exercises/

Neumann, M., Wirtz, M., Bollschweiler, E., Mercer, S.W., Warm, M., Wolf, J., & Pfaff, H. (2007). Determinants and patient-reported long-term outcomes of physician empathy in oncology: A structural equation modelling approach. *Patient Education and Counseling, 69*(1), 63–75. https://doi.org/10.1016/j.pec.2007.07.003

Paul-Savoie, E., Bourgault, P., Potvin, S., Gosselin, E., & Lafrenaye, S. (2018). The impact of pain invisibility on patient-centered care and empathetic attitude in chronic pain management. *Pain Research and Management, 2018*, e6375713. https://doi.org/10.1155/2018/6375713

Prosko, S. (2019). Compassion in Pain Care. In N. Pearson, S. Prosko, & M. Sullivan (eds) *Yoga and Science in Pain Care: Treating the Person in Pain.* (pp.235–256). London: Singing Dragon Publishers.

Ramsden, I.M. (2002). Cultural Safety and Nursing Education in Aotearoa and Te Waipounamu [Doctor of Philosophy in Nursing]. Victoria University of Wellington.

Rubak, S., Sandbæk, A., Lauritzen, T., & Christensen, B. (2005). Motivational interviewing: A systematic review and meta-analysis. *British Journal of General Practice*, *55*(513), 305–312.

Santana, M.J., Manalili, K., Jolley, R.J., Zelinsky, S., Quan, H., & Lu, M. (2018). How to practice person-centred care: A conceptual framework. *Health Expectations*, *21*(2), 429–440. https://doi.org/10.1111/hex.12640

Seppälä, E.M., Hutcherson, C.A., Nguyen, D.T., Doty, J.R., & Gross, J.J. (2014). Loving-kindness meditation: A tool to improve healthcare provider compassion, resilience, and patient care. *Journal of Compassionate Health Care*, *1*(1), 5. https://doi.org/10.1186/s40639-014-0005-9

Seppälä, E.M., Simon-Thomas, E., Brown, S.L., Worline, M.C., Cameron, C.D., & Doty, J.R. (eds) (2017). *The Oxford Handbook of Compassion Science, 1st edition*. Oxford: Oxford University Press.

Skolarus, T.A., Wolf, A.M.D., Erb, N.L., *et al.* (2014). American Cancer Society prostate cancer survivorship care guidelines. *CA: A Cancer Journal for Clinicians, 64*(4), 225–249. https://doi.org/10.3322/caac.21234

Smith, R.C., Fortin, A.H., Dwamena, F., & Frankel, R.M. (2013). An evidence-based patient-centered method makes the biopsychosocial model scientific. *Patient Education and Counseling, 91*(3), 265–270. https://doi.org/10.1016/j.pec.2012.12.010

Stilwell, P., & Harman, K. (2019). An Enactive Approach to Pain: Beyond the Biopsychosocial Model. *Phenomenology and the Cognitive Sciences, 18*(4), 637–665. https://doi.org/10.1007/s11097-019-09624-7

Sylvestro, H.M., Mobley, K., & Wester, K. (2021). Biopsychosocial models in cancer care: Application of a counseling model of wellness. *Journal of Counselor Leadership and Advocacy, 8*(2), 116–129. https://doi.org/10.1080/2326716X.2021.1946665

Thomas, T., Althouse, A., Sigler, L., Arnold, R., *et al.* (2021). Stronger therapeutic alliance is associated with better quality of life among patients with advanced cancer. *Psycho-Oncology, 30*(7), 1086–1094. https://doi.org/10.1002/pon.5648

Treasure, J. (2004). Motivational interviewing. *Advances in Psychiatric Treatment, 10*(5), 331–337. https://doi.org/10.1192/apt.10.5.331

Vapiwala, N., Miller, D., Laventure, B., Woodhouse, K., *et al.* (2021). Stigma, beliefs and perceptions regarding prostate cancer among Black and Latino men and women. *BMC Public Health, 21*(1), 758. https://doi.org/10.1186/s12889-021-10793-x

Vo, J.B., Gillman, A., Mitchell, K., & Nolan, T.S. (2021). Health disparities: Impact of health disparities and treatment decision-making biases on cancer adverse effects among Black cancer survivors. *Clinical Journal of Oncology Nursing, 25*(5), 17–24. https://doi.org/10.1188/21.CJON.S1.17-24

Watts, S., Leydon, G., Birch, B., Prescott, P., Lai, L., Eardley, S., & Lewith, G. (2014). Depression and anxiety in prostate cancer: A systematic review and meta-analysis of prevalence rates. *BMJ Open, 4*(3), e003901. https://doi.org/10.1136/bmjopen-2013-003901

Zhao, X., Sun, M., & Yang, Y. (2021). Effects of social support, hope and resilience on depressive symptoms within 18 months after diagnosis of prostate cancer. *Health and Quality of Life Outcomes, 19*(1), 15. https://doi.org/10.1186/s12955-020-01660-1

CHAPTER 6

The Bio Part 1: Pelvic Floor Rehabilitation and Bladder Training

I believe that the pelvis is a very emotional area in the human body: for example, it responds to triggers, emotions, and stress. Therefore, anyone who treats the pelvis needs to be attentive and to focus on the entire human being who owns the pelvis.

As previously discussed in Part One, biological changes may occur in the urinary and reproductive male systems, resulting in bladder, bowel, and sexual symptoms before, during, and after prostate cancer treatments. Some of these symptoms can be addressed conservatively through pelvic floor rehabilitation and bladder training. This chapter will present recent research recommendations and an overview for the assessment and treatment of male pelvic floor and lower urinary tract symptoms. Although this chapter will focus on the function and biological impact on the urinary, gastro, and sexual systems, the principles of the humanistic biopsychosocial approach should not be forgotten, especially when treating the pelvis and the pelvic floor muscles.

PELVIC FLOOR REHABILITATION IN PROSTATE CANCER SURVIVORSHIP: IMPLICATIONS AND REVIEW

There is increasing evidence to support pelvic floor rehabilitation in managing side-effects of prostate cancer and prostate cancer treatments. More specifically, starting pelvic floor muscle training (PFMT) is now encourged before prostate surgery to improve urinary and sexual outcomes.[1, 2] It may also reduce stress urinary incontinence or active incontinence post-op.[3] Recently, the American Urology Association produced evidence-based guidelines recommending PFMT before prostatectomy surgery (grade C evidence) and immediately after catheter removal (grade B evidence).[4] It has

---

1   (Mungovan *et al.*, 2021)
2   (Nahon *et al.*, 2014)
3   (Szczygielska *et al.*, 2022)
4   (Sandhu *et al.*, 2019)

been suggested that external sphincter tonus may contribute to prostatectomy urinary incontinence (PUI). Additionally, the levator ani muscles may facilitate increased posterior urethral compression, further supporting the case for pelvic floor muscle training as a treatment for PUI.

The heterogeneity of how continence is described in the literature and the variety of PFMT protocols and timing of intervention to date still present challenges for determining the best intervention for this population. Furthermore, considering the pathophysiology of PUI reviewed in Chapter 3, which suggests that passive incontinence may also be present, strengthening the striated muscles of the pelvic floor may not affect the compromised autonomic nervous system and smooth muscles of the urethra that result from surgery. Hence, a one-size-fits-all intervention for this population may not be appropriate.

Another factor to consider when prescribing PFMT to this population is that the physiology of male continence mechanisms may differ from females. Recent real-time ultrasound studies were able to include the role of the bulbospongiosus muscle in constricting the urethra to maintain urinary continence. These studies demonstrated that the bulbospongiosus compresses the urethra distally (dorsal to ventral) in opposition to the striated urethral sphincter (ventral to dorsal), and that they are activated first during increased intra-abdominal pressure.[5, 6] It was also demonstrated that puborectalis shortening may not correlate with return to continence post prostatectomy, so focusing on puborectalis training may not be effective for this population.[7] These implications may need to be considered when training the pelvic floor muscles, for example by teaching activation of these anterior muscles with possible cueing techniques that may differ from cueing techniques that will initiate only puborectalis contractions or anal striated sphincter muscles. Prompts such as "shorten the penis" and "stop the flow of urine" may be more efficacious (to optimize dorsal urethral displacement and striated urinary sphincter activation), than "tighten around the anus."[8]

There are only a few studies to date looking at PFMT for erectile function (EF) in prostate survivors; however, all the studies relate to those who had prostatectomy surgery.[9] The recommendations for treating erectile dysfunction in prostate cancer patients are still based on medical treatments, including prescription for pumps, medication, and intracavernosal injections.[10] Geraerts and colleagues' study demonstrated that PFMT may improve

5   (Stafford *et al.*, 2012)
6   (Hodges *et al.*, 2020)
7   (Neumann & O'Callaghan, 2018)
8   (Stafford *et al.*, 2016)
9   (Milios *et al.*, 2020)
10   (Shabataev *et al.*, 2020)

nerve-sparing prostatectomy erectile function and climacturia of those over 12 months of surgery.[11]

There is *no* study published to date on pelvic floor rehabilitation for improving bowel function of prostate cancer survivors. Fecal incontinence (FI) can be a side-effect of prostate radiation that can immensely impact prostate survivors' quality of life.[12] There is grade C evidence that PFMT can be efficacious in treating FI in the general population.[13] According to the few studies evaluating possible causes for FI post radiation therapy, some of the potential changes post radiation to the rectum are decreased external anal sphincter (EAS) squeezing and resting pressure and decreased rectal volume threshold during urge.[14] Increasing EAS strength, coordination, and tone through a pelvic rehabilitation program may be appropriate to help this population gain fecal control; however, studies in this area are needed to fill this *huge gap* in research.

Given that PFMT is non-invasive, and may potentially improve EF, UI, and FI, which are important prostate cancer survivorship issues, prescribing PFMT to prostate cancer survivors may be indicated. Timing of intervention can also be a factor, especially to reduce UI post-surgically and to see erectile function improvements in later stages of recovery. Moreover, the recruitment approaches should also be considered, as certain verbal cueing may facilitate contractions of the more ventral (anterior) part of the pelvic floor musculature compared to other verbal cueing.

PELVIC FLOOR MUSCLE ASSESSMENT

Currently there is no gold standard to assessing pelvic floor muscles, especially in males.[15] Recent studies have suggested that real-time ultrasound can be more reliable than digital rectal examination (DRE) when assessing rapid contractions and sustained-endurance pelvic floor muscles tests.[16] However, clinicians may still find DRE useful to evaluate the pelvic floor muscles' ability to contract and relax, as well as to assess tissue integrity and sensitivity.

The objective for this section is to provide novel insights of the male pelvic exam aligning to recent evidence provided in previous chapters. However, it is fundamental that physiotherapists and health professionals are suitably trained in the area of the male pelvic floor and practicing within their scope of practice, before attempting to evaluate the male pelvic floor and performing a digital rectal exam.

---

11 (Geraerts *et al.*, 2016)
12 (Damon *et al.*, 2008)
13 (Norton *et al.*, 2010)
14 (Maeda *et al.*, 2011)
15 (ICS Committees, 2018)
16 (Milios *et al.*, 2018)

INFORMED CONSENT

Regulatory bodies outline the importance in providing *informed consent* before medical treatment and examinations, particularly when performing a pelvic exam. The patient should be informed of the process, the risks, and benefits, and offered other forms of treatment and evaluation if available. Informed consent is at the center of patient–clinician therapeutic relationships.[17] As discussed in Chapter 5, fostering patient–clinician mutual trust and safety is fundamental for building a strong therapeutic alliance, especially in the area of pelvic health. Individuals should feel empowered during their interactions with their health professionals; and understanding that they can decline any treatment or examination that they don't feel comfortable doing should be the essence of the patient–clinician relationship.

Surface anatomy and digital rectal examination

As discussed in Chapter 2, the anatomy of the male pelvic floor differs from the female anatomy. It is important to note the landmarks of the male pelvis in order to evaluate the pelvic floor muscles and fascia system through palpation. Many studies suggest the importance of initially learning to activate the pelvic floor muscles without co-contracting abdominals, and gluteus and leg adductor muscles, ideally enhancing urethra closure without increasing intra-abdominal pressure.[18] This "technique" and efficacy of the patient's pelvic floor muscle contraction can be observed initially through perineal examination. A "shorten the penis" prompt may help to activate bulbospongiosus contraction, and "tighten around the anus" may help to activate external anal sphincter.[19] Bulbospongiosus, ischiocavernosus, and external anal sphincter can be palpated through perineal exam as demonstrated in Figure 6.1.

Carriere and Feldt suggested that it is possible to differentiate between the pelvic floor muscles when assessing their contractions during vaginal digital palpation in females: for example, distinguishing between a cranial–ventral movement facilitated by the puborectalis muscles, a cranial and medial movement from possibly the most anterior portion of the pubococcygeus and the elevation of the bladder neck when placing the finger behind the urethra.[20] However, no published literature was found on pelvic floor muscle modes of digital examination in males to differentiate between puborectalis and other

17   (Copnell, 2018)
18   (Stafford *et al.*, 2016)
19   (Stafford *et al.*, 2016)
20   (Carriere & Feldt, 2006)

pelvic floor muscles. Clinically, it may be possible to differentiate between the different pelvic floor muscle activations during DRE. For example, during DRE the puborectalis muscle contraction, a dorsal–ventral displacement can be palpated at the 6 o'clock mark at approximately 2–3 inches deep. The ventral–dorsal displacement of the EUS can be palpated at the 1–2 o'clock and 10–11 o'clock marks directly behind the pubic bone.

Male perineum surface anatomy

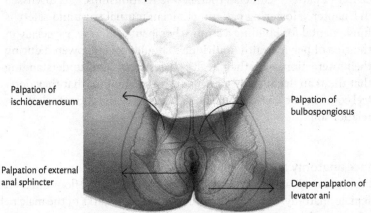

Palpation of
ischiocavernosum

Palpation of
bulbospongiosus

Palpation of external
anal sphincter

Deeper palpation of
levator ani

FIGURE 6.1: SUPERFICIAL PALPATION OF THE PERINEAL AND LEVATOR ANI MUSCLES

Ultrasound imaging

Transabdominal ultrasound imaging

Transabdominal ultrasound imaging (TrAUS), when positioned directly superior to the pubic bone, can show a cranial displacement of the bladder base during a puborectalis contraction.[21] It can be a non-invasive form of pelvic floor muscle assessment, and was shown to have high inter- and intra-rater reliability.[22] The cranial displacement of the bladder base is associated with a PFM contraction assessed via DRE, but weaker contractions palpated via DRE may not be well identified via TrAUS.[23] Images will be less clear of those who are unable to hold a significant amount of urine due to urine leakage.[24]

PROCEDURE

The curvilinear probe is placed on a transverse orientation above the pubic bone across the midline of the abdomen, aiming the transducer to about 60 degrees from vertical towards the bladder base. The transducer angulation

---

21 (Nahon *et al.*, 2011)
22 (Milios *et al.*, n.d.)
23 (Nahon *et al.*, 2011)
24 (Nahon *et al.*, 2011)

may vary according to the individual's body shape.[25] The common marker used to calculate the bladder displacement is in the region of the posterior-inferior bladder wall (Figure 6.2).[26] The individual can be assessed in supine, sitting, or standing positions; however, it is recommended that assessments be standardized, as bladder displacement can differ between crook-lying and standing positions.[27] It is recommended to standardize the bladder filling protocol, as the posterior–inferior bladder wall is best observed with a moderately full bladder. For example, the patient can be asked to empty the bladder one hour before the assessment time and then drink about 500ml of water after urination.[28]

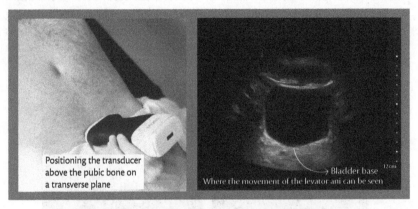

FIGURE 6.2: TRANSABDOMINAL ULTRASOUND IMAGING OF
THE BLADDER: TRANSDUCER POSITION AND IMAGE

Transperineal ultrasound imaging

Transperineal ultrasound imaging (TrPUS) may show some benefits in assessing the male pelvic floor muscles as it provides the visualization of the pubic bone as a bony landmark and the entire urethral length.[29] Through TrPUS, the three possible male urinary-continent striated muscles can be identified via displacement of the urethral–vesical junction (two landmarks), the anorectal angle, the bulb of penis, and mid-urethra.[30] These five landmarks are represented in Figure 6.3.

- UVJ1 & UVJ2: The cranial-ventral displacement of the urethral-vesical junction.

25 (Nahon *et al.*, 2011)
26 (Whittaker *et al.*, 2007)
27 (Kelly *et al.*, 2007)
28 (Whittaker *et al.*, 2007)
29 (Stafford *et al.*, 2012)
30 (Stafford *et al.*, 2012)

- ARJ: The anorectal angle corresponding to the levator ani contraction (puborectalis).
- BP: The bulb of penis dorsal to ventral displacement corresponding to bulbospongiosus contraction.
- MU: The ventral to dorsal displacement of the mid-urethra corresponding to the EUS contraction.[31]

PROCEDURE

In order to identify the five landmarks representing the striated urinary continence muscles, the curvilinear *covered* probe is placed on a mid-sagittal plane over the perineal body, midway between the scrotum and the anus. The individual can be assessed semi-reclined with knees bent or in standing (Figure 6.4). Bladder filling helps to facilitate the landmark identifications as the bladder image will be clearer; however, it is possible to identify the five landmarks without a full bladder.

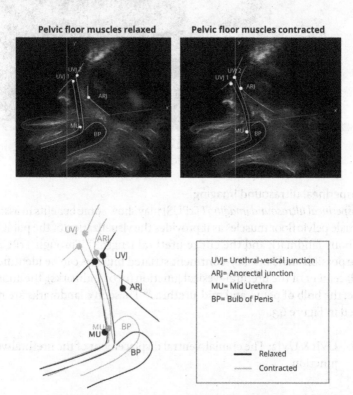

FIGURE 6.3: LANDMARKS AND DISPLACEMENTS OF THE
MALE STRIATED URINARY CONTINENCE MUSCLES
Adapted and modified from Stafford et al., 2012[32]

31   (Hodges *et al.*, 2020)
32   (Stafford *et al.*, 2012)

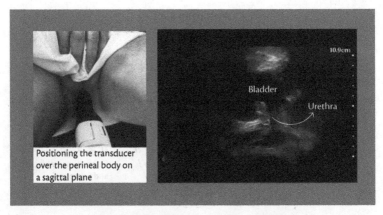

FIGURE 6.4: TRANSPERINEAL ULTRASOUND IMAGING OF THE
BLADDER: TRANSDUCER POSITION AND IMAGE

Biofeedback with surface EMG

Biofeedback with surface EMG on the anal sphincter, or on the bulbospongiosus muscles, can provide guidance to clinicians and patients regarding anal sphincter, puborectalis, and bulbospongiosus contraction and relaxation. However, it won't give information on the EUS contractions.[33] As a more invasive type of EMG, rectal EMG probes can also be used as another form of biofeedback and have been shown to possibly record and aggregate activities from the anterior and posterior levator ani muscles, the external anal sphincter, the bulbospongiosus, and ischiocavernosus muscles.[34] The PFM activity at rest and the ability to relax after contractions may be easier to identify using surface EMG technology.[35] It can be a less expensive method of biofeedback compared to ultrasound imaging, but the technology limitations need to be taken in consideration when using it as an assessment tool. Electromyography signals may be influenced by body posture, electrode type, and inter-electrode distance,[36] and may be susceptible to "crosstalk" from nearby muscles.[37] Figure 6.5 illustrates examples of surface EMG placements.

---

33 (Hodges *et al.*, 2020)
34 (Yani *et al.*, 2022)
35 (Yani *et al.*, 2022)
36 (Roman-Liu, 2016)
37 (Auchincloss & McLean, 2009)

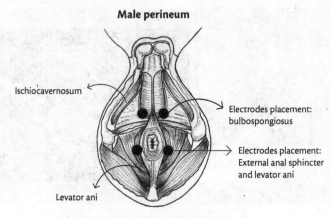

FIGURE 6.5: SURFACE EMG PLACEMENTS

Table 6.1: Comparison of methods for evaluating the pelvic floor muscles (PFM)

Method	Pros	Cons
Digital rectal exam (DRE)	• Low cost • Can be integrated with tissue and relaxation evaluation • May be able to identify weaker PFM contractions	• Invasive • May not be indicated for individuals with trauma history • Has not shown to be as reliable as TrAUS or TrPUS[38]
Transabdominal US (TrAUS)	• Minimizes discomfort and embarrassment • Shown to be valid and reliable[39] • May require less training than TrPUS	• Bladder needs to be full • No fixed point of reference • Does not evaluate all PFM • May not identify weaker PFM contractions[40] • Expensive
Transperineal US (TrPUS)	• Has a fixed point of reference • Able to visualize the entire urethra • Able to evaluate all PFM • Less invasive than DRE • Urethra can be visualized with an empty bladder • Reliable	• Patient still needs to undress • Clinician may need to be more experienced, or have increased training • Expensive

38 (Milios et al., 2018)
39 (Nahon et al., 2011)
40 (Nahon et al., 2011)

Surface EMG	<ul><li>May be a good form of visual biofeedback for patients</li><li>Sticker form is less invasive than DRE</li><li>More cost effective than US</li><li>May be easier to identify increased PFM activity at rest or after PFM contractions[41]</li></ul>	<ul><li>Not able to assess the EUS</li><li>May record "cross-talk" from other nearby muscles[42]</li><li>Patients still need to disrobe</li><li>Recordings may be influenced by body posture, electrode type, inter-electrode distance[43]</li><li>Rectal probes can be as invasive as DRE</li></ul>

PELVIC FLOOR MUSCLE TRAINING (PFMT)
Novel pelvic floor rehabilitation proposed for post-prostatectomy urinary incontinence

A recently published article proposed a different approach to pelvic floor rehabilitation pertaining to those with urinary incontinence after prostatectomy surgery.[44] According to Hodges and colleagues, the emphasis should be in training the anterior striated continence muscles (bulbospongiosus and EUS) while minimizing puborectalis muscle engagement. Their protocol encourages pre-op and post-op rehabilitation, principles of pelvic floor muscles motor learning mostly biased to the EUS, using transperineal ultrasound imaging for patient's assessment, and biofeedback, while focusing on function rather than strictly muscle strengthening. Their proposed PFM assessments will involve a series of functional tasks to tailor each individual's training focus. The ultimate goal would be to integrate PFMT into functional tasks, for example training pre-activation before exertion or maintaining low intensity PFM holds for longer periods of time. Currently, there is a randomized control trial being conducted to test this novel training approach, which is expected to be published at the end of 2023.

Jo Milios and colleagues showed that a different protocol of PFMT pre-op targeting both slow and fast twitch fibers demonstrated a faster return to continence compared to a protocol more focused on slow twitch fibers. This protocol consisted of six sets of 10 fast contractions (1 sec each), and 10 slow contractions (10 sec contraction and 10 sec relaxation) six times daily,

---

41 (Yani *et al.*, 2022)
42 (Auchincloss & McLean, 2009)
43 (Roman-Liu, 2016)
44 (Hodges *et al.*, 2020)

performing in a standing posture. The cues used to facilitate PFM contraction were "Stop the flow of urine and shorten the penis."[45]

Other types of program can include:

- *The "knack,"* which is training PFM contraction before coughing and sneezing.
- *Milking technique,* which incorporates a PFM contraction after urination to help expel urine from the urethra and eliminate post-void UI.
- *PFMT with core activation*, which has also been used to improve core muscles co-contraction activities; for example, training transverse abdominal muscle activation after pelvic floor muscle contraction during a leg lift exercise may help those who have poor core control and are at risk for abdominal hernias post-op.
- *PFMT progressions*, such as adding PFM contraction with increased load (e.g., using weights), with posture variations (e.g., progressing from a lying position, to sitting, to standing, to squatting etc.), and during functional activity (e.g., adding PFM endurance training during the first 5–10 minutes of a walking program, or a PFM strength training program during the first 5–10 minutes of a weight training program).

Table 6.2: Example of how to progress PFMT

Easiest ←——————————————————————————————→ Hardest

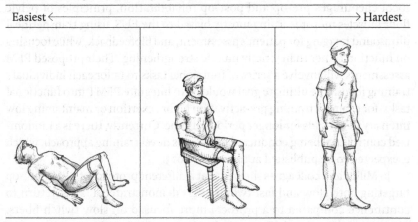

PFMT and urgency

Although the literature still remains inconclusive regarding PFMT being effective in reducing symptoms of overactive bladder (OAB), such as urgency and frequency,[46] it may still be relevant in clinical settings to assess and treat pelvic floor muscle dysfunction in prostate cancer survivors with symptoms

---

45   (Milios *et al.*, 2019)
46   (Monteiro *et al.*, 2018)

of OAB. For example, it has been shown that neuromuscular education and interval bladder training in males with symptoms of chronic prostate pain syndrome (including biofeedback using surface EMG) helped to reduce urgency and voiding frequency.[47] Also, combination of PFMT and behavioral therapy seemed to be more effective in reducing urge UI compared to other forms of treatment such as behavioral therapy alone, PFMT alone, or drug therapy.[48] Clinically, there *may* be an association with pelvic floor tension and symptoms of urgency and frequency, so when thinking of prescribing PFMT for this population, clinicians may need to be cautious, and assess pelvic floor relaxation and tension before and throughout the program.

PFMT and FI

As mentioned previously, PFMT *may* improve fecal incontinence in prostate cancer survivors.[49] Before recommending pelvic floor rehabilitation to this population, the external and internal anal sphincter muscles should be assessed. According to the assessment findings and if appropriate, a program more focused on the posterior part of the levator ani muscles and the EAS should be prescribed. Prompts such as "tighten around the anus" or "stopping gas," may be more effective in facilitating the contraction of the posterior pelvic floor muscles.

PFMT for ED and climacturia

PFMT can be beneficial to improve penile hardness, length, tumescence, and elevation, as well as climacturia for nerve-sparing prostatectomy patients. According to Geraerts and colleagues' study, a three-month PFMT home program of 60 contractions per day spread over two sessions, focusing on strength, endurance, coordination, and dual task combination, was shown to improve ED and urinary incontinence during orgasm in patients at a *minimum of 12 months after radical prostatectomy.* This study's home program was facilitated by six initial weeks of weekly sessions and then sessions every 14 days, with a pelvic floor therapist, supported by electro stimulation (biphasic symmetrical current, intensity as high as possible, not painful, frequency of 50 Hz, and pulse duration of 600 μs).[50] However, this study did not specify the particular pelvic floor muscles that were targeted or the electrode placements used during stimulation. It remains unclear whether the rehabilitation included the ischiocavernosus and bulbospongiosus muscles, which are important for sustaining penile erection. When developing a treatment plan to enhance sexual function, it could be advantageous to incorporate the rehabilitation of muscles involved in maintaining penile erection, such as the ischiocavernosus and bulbospongiosus muscles.

---

47 (Clemens *et al.*, 2000)
48 (Reisch, 2020)
49 (Norton *et al.*, 2010)
50 (Geraerts *et al.*, 2016)

PELVIC FLOOR RELAXATION

Pelvic floor relaxation training can also help those with pelvic floor muscles that are tensed or overactive, or who have difficulties with relaxation, and may be a good starting point in training the pelvic floor (especially for those still experiencing pain post-op). A more tailored prescription of pelvic floor interventions based on pelvic floor physical examination findings may be more appropriate for treating pelvic floor dysfunction when addressing bladder, bowel, and sexual concerns of prostate cancer survivors. A recent retrospective chart review of 136 patients with post-prostatectomy urinary incontinence treated with a tailored pelvic floor physiotherapy, including using relaxation techniques for overactive pelvic floor, was shown to reduce UI and pelvic pain post-surgery.[51] Patients with overactive pelvic floor dysfunction were provided guidance on a "downtraining" program that focused on promoting relaxation. This program included techniques such as diaphragmatic breathing, stretches, and perineal bulges, also known as reverse Kegels, which is a training technique that incorporates diaphragmatic breathing with pelvic-floor muscle relaxation and lengthening (during inhalation). Additionally, manual therapy was incorporated as part of the treatment, involving external and intrarectal myofascial release to alleviate trigger points, lengthen tissues, and mobilize scar tissue. Patients with an overactive pelvic floor were not instructed in Kegel exercises or any other strengthening exercises.[52]

While there may be limited research specifically investigating pelvic floor relaxation for prostate cancer survivors, who tend to brace and contract their pelvic floor muscles in response to emotional triggers or fear about urinary leakages, the concept of utilizing relaxation techniques in such situations can still be beneficial.

Prostate cancer survivors often experience various emotional and psychological challenges as they navigate the post-treatment phase. Anxiety, fear, and worry about urinary leakage or other pelvic floor issues may lead to increased muscle tension and involuntary contractions of the pelvic floor muscles. This constant bracing and contraction can further exacerbate pelvic floor dysfunction. Van Lunsen and Ramakers suggested that traumatic experiences, somatization, and anxiety disorders may result in muscle tension and pelvic floor hyperactivity.[53] They also suggested that the coexistence of pelvic floor complaints, anxiety disorders, somatization, and traumatic experiences indicates a harmful cycle where pelvic floor hyperactivity, psychological disorders, and physical symptoms reinforce one another.[54]

In this context, pelvic floor relaxation techniques can be helpful. By consciously focusing on relaxing the pelvic floor muscles, individuals can learn

51   (Scott *et al.*, 2020)
52   (Scott *et al.*, 2020)
53   (Van Lunsen & Ramakers, 2002)
54   (Van Lunsen & Ramakers, 2002)

to release tension and reduce the habit of bracing. Deep breathing exercises, visualization, progressive muscle relaxation, and mindfulness techniques are examples of relaxation methods that can be incorporated into a pelvic floor relaxation routine. Reverse Kegel exercises can also be incorporated into a program, counterbalancing strength training programs. Biofeedback using EMG or Real Time Ultrasound can be used too as pelvic floor relaxation teaching tools. Lengthening of the pelvic floor can additionally be encouraged by pelvic "opening" postures, such as the yoga pose "Happy Baby," perineal pose, modified butterfly pose, or symmetry pose, and wall straddle pose. These postures can be sustained for a longer period of time while incorporating relaxation breathing techniques.

While specific studies on this aspect may be lacking, the general principles of relaxation and its potential benefits for managing muscle tension and emotional triggers are widely recognized. Engaging in pelvic floor relaxation exercises can promote a sense of calmness, reduce muscle tension, and enhance overall pelvic floor function. These techniques can contribute to a greater sense of control and improved emotional wellbeing, and potentially help manage urinary leakage and related concerns in prostate cancer survivors.

Opening poses

All of these poses are intended to promote relaxation, so the sensations experienced during these stretches should not be overly intense. To maximize the benefits, it is recommended to spend a minimum of two minutes in each pose, allowing ample time for the body to fully relax and benefit from the stretch.

Symmetry pose or reclined butterfly

This pose was shown to be the most beneficial in providing pelvic floor muscle relaxation.[55] Lie on your back with your knees bent, bringing the soles of your feet together. If needed, utilize additional support such as pillows or props to find a comfortable position. Take a moment to observe any sensations of pain, stretch, or potential asymmetry in your body.

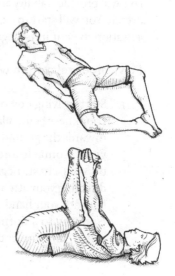

The Happy Baby pose: Ananda Balasana

Bring your bent knees towards your chest, keep the feet flexed, and bring the knees wider than your torso, allowing them to fall towards your

---

55   (Tosun *et al.*, 2022)

armpits. Your thighs should be perpendicular to the floor. Reach your arms through the inside of your thighs and hold onto the outside edges of your feet or grab your ankles. If you can't reach your feet, you can also hold onto your shins or use a strap around the feet.

As you hold onto your feet or ankles, gently pull them downwards, encouraging your knees to move closer towards the floor.

Relax your shoulders and lengthen your neck, allowing your head to rest comfortably on the ground.

Perineal pose

Sit against a wall or a bed headboard, utilizing pillows if necessary to achieve a semi-reclined position. Bend your knees, bringing them closer to your thighs, and separate your feet wider than your hips. Open your knees wide and consciously relax the muscles of the pelvic floor.

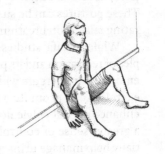

Wall straddle pose

Find an open wall space and sit sideways to the wall, ensuring your seat is as close to the wall as possible. Rotate your body so that you are facing the wall while lying on your back. Gently bring your legs up the wall, allowing them to open as far as feels comfortable. If you are less flexible, you can keep your knees bent. Make sure your pelvis is well supported by the wall, ensuring there is no gap between the wall and your pelvis. This will provide stability and support during the stretch. You will start to experience a stretching sensation in your inner legs.

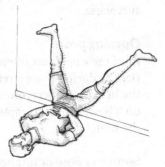

Pelvic floor relaxation with diaphragmatic breathing

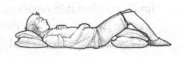

1. Start by lying down on your back with your knees bent, relaxing your tailbone towards the ground. Place one hand on your stomach and the other hand on your chest. Begin this exercise by directing your attention to your breath and observing the movements beneath your hands. Begin to gradually slow down your breathing by counting to 4 during inhalation and 6 during exhalation. Placing a rolled towel under the sacrum can help encourage a posture of pelvic relaxation.

2. Change your breathing pattern by allowing your abdomen to expand while keeping your chest still. Visualize a colored balloon just below your belly button and imagine it expanding up and down with each inhalation. Use this opportunity to relax your abdominal muscles. As you inhale, let your abdominal muscles relax, allowing 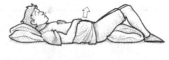 the abdominal wall to expand and your pelvic floor muscles to relax and lengthen. Avoid forcing or bearing down while breathing. Simply visualize the air reaching deeper with each breath.

3. Exhale slowly, while keeping your abdominal muscles relaxed. Imagine gently opening the neck of the balloon and allowing the air to escape without any strain or force.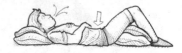

OTHER INFLUENCERS: BREATHING AND PRESSURE

It may be relevant to incorporate training of PFM synergistic muscles of the abdominopelvic cavity and the thoracic diaphragm, as they contribute to controlling intra-abdominal pressure (IAP). Physiologically, the three-layered anterolateral abdominal muscles (external oblique, internal oblique, and transverse abdominis) and the rectus abdominis, the PFM, and the thoracic diaphragm and the glottis modulate IAP.[56] According to a study by Niederauer and colleagus, elevated intra-abdominal pressure is most strongly correlated with hip acceleration, volume of respiration, and moments of abdominal and thoracic flexion.[57] Training programs that focus on effective strategies to decrease intra-abdominal pressure (IAP) during tasks that trigger urinary incontinence (UI)—for example, employing breathing and movement techniques to decrease inspiration volumes and hip acceleration, while facilitating pelvic floor muscle activation and synergistic muscle contractions (such as diaphragmatic activation)—may result in a reduction of IAP and improvement in functional goals.

Decreasing IAP during a sit-to-stand exercise:

Before standing up, move forward on the chair and place one foot behind the other while keeping the other foot slightly forward. Take a slow and deep breath in, and as you exhale, stand up with a tall and upright posture, without excessively bending the hip. Use your legs to push yourself up, rather than relying on your arms, and avoid tensing your upper body or bearing down

---

56 (Talasz *et al.*, 2022)
57 (Niederauer *et al.*, 2022)

while standing up. Make the task as easy and effortless as possible. Once standing, take a moment before beginning to walk.

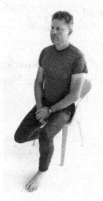	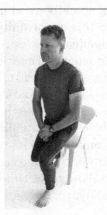
1) Preparation for standing	2) Inhale as you shift forward in the chair and move one leg forward while moving the other leg back
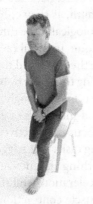	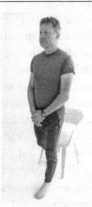
3) Exhale to stand up using the leg muscles and not pushing down with the arms	4) Wait a few seconds before moving and allow the bladder to adjust to the new posture

BEHAVIORAL THERAPY AND BLADDER TRAINING

It is recommended as level 1B-2 evidence for those with lower urinary tract symptoms, such as urgency and frequency, to adopt lifestyle changes and bladder habits that may contribute to lower urinary tract symptoms.

- Reduction in caffeine can improve frequency, urgency, and UI.[58]

---

58 (Tse *et al.*, 2016)

- Increase in fluid intake may not be associated with increased urine loss.[59]
- Reduction in weight can improve UI and OAB symptoms.[60]
- Bowel habits, such as improving stool consistency and having regular bowel movements which are easy to pass, can reduce urinary urgency.[61]
- Bladder training, which includes following a voiding schedule with timed intervals of 2.5 to 4 hours, or deferring urination until the strong urge "settles," may improve urgency and frequency.[62]
- Urge suppression techniques, for example, sitting down, practicing quick voluntary pelvic floor muscle contractions, and distracting the mind after strong urge occurs, can reduce frequency and urgency.[63]

BLADDER TRAINING POST-PROSTATECTOMY: A PROPOSED THEORY TO HELP REGAIN URINARY CONTROL

Having been treating this population for over 13 years, I noticed that over-urination may delay urinary control. Most men after surgery who "over"-urinate may do so to compensate and try to avoid urinary incontinence. The theory is that accumulating urine in the bladder may help neurological urinary control and sympathetic response. For example, detrusor muscle relaxation may encourage urethral smooth muscle contraction. The "weight" of a filled bladder may also encourage the external urethral sphincter type-1 slow-twitch fiber activation.

You may coach your patients to start urinating every two hours and slowly start to increase the time between urination as control starts to improve. Urge suppression techniques can be applied to reduce urge while spacing time between urination.

For those who are unable to retain urine while standing, you can encourage them to sit or lie down for a few hours during the day in order to accumulate some urine in their bladder. Adjusting their sleeping habits can also help bladder training: for example, decreasing the amount of times they wake up to urinate in the middle of the night can help improve bladder filling during the night, and improve urination flow and volume in the mornings when they wake up.

---

59   (Tomlinson *et al.*, 1999)
60   (Tse *et al.*, 2016)
61   (Alhababi *et al.*, 2021)
62   (Tse *et al.*, 2016)
63   (Pal *et al.*, 2021)

CONCLUSION

This chapter provides a review and discussion of the supporting evidence for pelvic floor rehabilitation in treating bladder, bowel, and sexual symptoms of prostate cancer survivors. It also discusses some novel theories and approaches that may address symptoms arising after treatment. A more intense pre-operative program, which includes fast and slow twitch pelvic floor muscle rehabilitation, seems to speed up recovery after prostatectomy surgery. Pelvic floor muscle assessments, such as transperineal ultrasound or a focused digital rectal exam, may help to identify the three possible urethral striated muscles responsible for controlling urinary continence in males. However, other forms of pelvic floor assessments, such as surface EMG or transabdominal ultrasound, may need to be offered for patients who do not consent to a more invasive exam. Prompts such as "shorten the penis" or "stop the flow of urine" may help to facilitate the bulbospongiosus and external urethral sphincter contractions, and *"tighten around the anus"* may better facilitate the external anal sphincter and puborectalis muscles. Bladder training and behavioral changes may also improve lower urinary tract symptoms, including urgency, frequency, and possibly urinary incontinence. There is still a significant gap in the literature regarding conservative treatments (including PFMT, bladder training, and pelvic floor relaxation) for prostate cancer survivors who experience bladder, bowel, and sexual dysfunction. Most of the current research on conservative treatments is only related to prostatectomy survivors, excluding a large population of prostate cancer survivors.

REFERENCES

Alhababi, N., Magnus, M.C., Drake, M.J., Fraser, A., & Joinson, C. (2021). The association between constipation and lower urinary tract symptoms in parous middle-aged women: A prospective cohort study. *Journal of Women's Health (15409996)*, *30*(8), 1171–1181. https://doi.org/10.1089/jwh.2020.8624

Auchincloss, C.C., & McLean, L. (2009). Simultaneous recordings of surface and fine-wire pelvic floor muscle EMG. *Physiotherapy Canada*, *61*, 41–42.

Carriere, B., & Feldt, C.M. (eds) (2006). *The Pelvic Floor, 1st edition.* New York: Thieme.

Clemens, J.Q., Nadler, R.B., Schaeffer, A.J., Belani, J., Albaugh, J., & Bushman, W. (2000). Biofeedback, pelvic floor re-education, and bladder training for male chronic pelvic pain syndrome. *Urology*, *56*(6), 951–955. https://doi.org/10.1016/S0090-4295(00)00796-2

Copnell, G. (2018). Informed consent in physiotherapy practice: It is not what is said but how it is said. *Physiotherapy*, *104*(1), 67–71. https://doi.org/10.1016/j.physio.2017.07.006

Damon, H., Schott, A.M., Barth, X., Faucheron, J.L., *et al.* (2008). Clinical characteristics and quality of life in a cohort of 621 patients with faecal incontinence. *International Journal of Colorectal Disease*, *23*(9), 845–851. https://doi.org/10.1007/s00384-008-0489-x

Geraerts, I., Van Poppel, H., Devoogdt, N., De Groef, A., Fieuws, S., & Van Kampen, M. (2016). Pelvic floor muscle training for erectile dysfunction and climacturia 1 year after nerve sparing radical prostatectomy: A randomized controlled trial. *International Journal of Impotence Research*, *28*(1), Article 1. https://doi.org/10.1038/ijir.2015.24

Hodges, P.W., Stafford, R.E., Hall, L., Neumann, P., *et al.* (2020). Reconsideration of pelvic floor muscle training to prevent and treat incontinence after radical prostatectomy. *Urologic*

Oncology: Seminars and Original Investigations, 38(5), 354–371. https://doi.org/10.1016/j.urolonc.2019.12.007

ICS Committees (2018). *Digital Palpation of the Pelvic Floor Muscles.* Retrieved November 29, 2022, from https://www.ics.org/committees/standardisation/terminologydiscussions/digitalpalpationofthepelvicfloormuscles

Kelly, M., Tan, B.-K., Thompson, J., Carroll, S., Follington, M., Arndt, A., & Seet, M. (2007). Healthy adults can more easily elevate the pelvic floor in standing than in crook-lying: An experimental study. *Australian Journal of Physiotherapy, 53*(3), 187–191. https://doi.org/10.1016/S0004-9514(07)70026-0

Maeda, Y., Høyer, M., Lundby, L., & Norton, C. (2011). Faecal incontinence following radiotherapy for prostate cancer: A systematic review. *Radiotherapy and Oncology, 98*(2), 145–153. https://doi.org/10.1016/j.radonc.2010.12.004

Milios, J.E., Ackland, T.R., & Green, D.J. (2019). Pelvic floor muscle training in radical prostatectomy: A randomized controlled trial of the impacts on pelvic floor muscle function and urinary incontinence. *BMC Urology, 19*(1), 116. https://doi.org/10.1186/s12894-019-0546-5

Milios, J.E., Ackland, T.R., & Green, D.J. (2020). Pelvic floor muscle training and erectile dysfunction in radical prostatectomy: A randomized controlled trial investigating a non-invasive addition to penile rehabilitation. *Sexual Medicine, 8*(3), 414–421. https://doi.org/10.1016/j.esxm.2020.03.005

Milios, J.E., Atkinson, C.L., Naylor, L.H., Millar, D., Thijssen, D.H.J., Ackland, T.R., & Green, D.J. (2018). Pelvic floor muscle assessment in men post prostatectomy: Comparing digital rectal examination and real-time ultrasound approaches. *Australian & New Zealand Continence Journal, 24*(4), 105–111.

Monteiro, S., Riccetto, C., Araújo, A., Galo, L., Brito, N., & Botelho, S. (2018). Efficacy of pelvic floor muscle training in women with overactive bladder syndrome: A systematic review. *International Urogynecology Journal, 29*(11), 1565–1573. https://doi.org/10.1007/s00192-018-3602-x

Mungovan, S.F., Carlsson, S.V., Gass, G.C., Graham, P.L., *et al.* (2021). Preoperative exercise interventions to optimize continence outcomes following radical prostatectomy. *Nature Reviews Urology, 18*(5), 259–281. https://doi.org/10.1038/s41585-021-00445-5

Nahon, I., Waddington, G., Adams, R., & Dorey, G. (2011). Assessing muscle function of the male pelvic floor using real time ultrasound. *Neurourology and Urodynamics, 30*(7), 1329–1332. https://doi.org/10.1002/nau.21069

Nahon, I., Martin, M., & Adams, R. (2014). Pre-operative pelvic floor muscle training—A review. *Urologic Nursing, 34*(5), 230–237. https://doi.org/10.7257/1053-816X.2014.34.5.230

Neumann, P.B., & O'Callaghan, M. (2018). The role of preoperative puborectal muscle function assessed by transperineal ultrasound in urinary continence outcomes at 3, 6, and 12 months after robotic-assisted radical prostatectomy. *International Neurourology Journal, 22*(2), 114–122. https://doi.org/10.5213/inj.1836026.013

Niederauer, S., Hunt, G., Foreman, K.B., Merryweather, A., & Hitchcock, R. (2022). Intrinsic factors contributing to elevated intra-abdominal pressure. *Computer Methods in Biomechanics and Biomedical Engineering, 26*(8), 941–951. https://doi.org/10.1080/10255842.2022.2100220

Norton, C., Whitehead, W.E., Bliss, D.Z., Harari, D., & Lang, J. (2010). Management of fecal incontinence in adults. *Neurourology and Urodynamics, 29*(1), 199–206. https://doi.org/10.1002/nau.20803

Pal, M., Chowdhury, R., & Bandyopadhyay, S. (2021). Urge suppression and modified fluid consumption in the management of female overactive bladder symptoms. *Urology Annals, 13*(3), 263–267. https://doi.org/10.4103/UA.UA_52_20

Reisch, R. (2020). Interventions for overactive bladder: Review of pelvic floor muscle training and urgency control strategies. *Journal of Women's Health Physical Therapy, 44*(1), 19–25. https://doi.org/10.1097/JWH.0000000000000148

Roman-Liu, D. (2016). The influence of confounding factors on the relationship between muscle contraction level and MF and MPF values of EMG signal: A review. *International Journal of Occupational Safety and Ergonomics, 22*(1), 77–91. https://doi.org/10.1080/10803548.2015.1116817

Sandhu, J.S., Breyer, B., Comiter, C., Eastham, J.A., *et al.* (2019). Incontinence after prostate treatment: AUA/SUFU Guideline. *Journal of Urology*, *202*(2), 369–378. https://doi.org/10.1097/JU.0000000000000314

Scott, K.M., Gosai, E., Bradley, M.H., Walton, S., Hynan, L.S., Lemack, G., & Roehrborn, C. (2020). Individualized pelvic physical therapy for the treatment of post-prostatectomy stress urinary incontinence and pelvic pain. *International Urology and Nephrology*, *52*(4), 655–659. https://doi.org/10.1007/s11255-019-02343-7

Shabataev, V., Saadat, S.H., & Elterman, D.S. (2020). Management of erectile dysfunction and LUTS/incontinence: The two most common, long-term side-effects of prostate cancer treatment. *Canadian Journal of Urology*, *27*(27 Suppl 1), 17–24.

Stafford, R.E., Ashton-Miller, J.A., Constantinou, C.E., & Hodges, P.W. (2012). Novel insight into the dynamics of male pelvic floor contractions through transperineal ultrasound imaging. *Journal of Urology*, *188*(4), 1224–1230. https://doi.org/10.1016/j.juro.2012.06.028

Stafford, R.E., Ashton-Miller, J.A., Constantinou, C., Coughlin, G., Lutton, N.J., & Hodges, P.W. (2016). Pattern of activation of pelvic floor muscles in men differs with verbal instructions. *Neurourology and Urodynamics*, *35*(4), 457–463. https://doi.org/10.1002/nau.22745

Szczygielska, D., Knapik, A., Pop, T., Rottermund, J., & Saulicz, E. (2022). The effectiveness of pelvic floor muscle training in men after radical prostatectomy measured with the Insert Test. *International Journal of Environmental Research and Public Health*, *19*(5). https://doi.org/10.3390/ijerph19052890

Talasz, H., Kremser, C., Talasz, H.J., Kofler, M., & Rudisch, A. (2022). Breathing, (s)training and the pelvic floor—A basic concept. *Healthcare*, *10*(6), 1035. https://doi.org/10.3390/healthcare10061035

Tomlinson, B.U., Dougherty, M.C., Pendergast, J.F., Boyington, A.R., Coffman, M.A., & Pickens, S.M. (1999). Dietary caffeine, fluid intake and urinary incontinence in older rural women. *International Urogynecology Journal and Pelvic Floor Dysfunction*, *10*(1), 22–28. https://doi.org/10.1007/pl00004009

Tosun, Ö.Ç., Dayıcan, D.K., Keser, İ., Kurt, S., Yıldırım, M., & Tosun, G. (2022). Are clinically recommended pelvic floor muscle relaxation positions really efficient for muscle relaxation? *International Urogynecology Journal*, *33*(9), 2391–2400. https://doi.org/10.1007/s00192-022-05119-3

Tse, V., King, J., Dowling, C., English, S., *et al.* (2016). Conjoint Urological Society of Australia and New Zealand (USANZ) and Urogynaecological Society of Australasia (UGSA) Guidelines on the management of adult non-neurogenic overactive bladder. *BJU International*, *117*(1), 34–47. https://doi.org/10.1111/bju.13246

Van Lunsen, R.H.W., & Ramakers, M.J. (2002). Le syndrome du plancher pelvien hyperactif (SPPH). *Acta Endoscopica*, *32*(3), 275–285. https://doi.org/10.1007/BF03020230

Whittaker, J.L., Thompson, J.A., Teyhen, D.S., & Hodges, P. (2007). Rehabilitative ultrasound imaging of pelvic floor muscle function. *Journal of Orthopaedic & Sports Physical Therapy*, *37*(8), 487–498. https://doi.org/10.2519/jospt.2007.2548

Yani, M.S., Eckel, S.P., Kirages, D.J., Rodriguez, L.V., Corcos, D.M., & Kutch, J.J. (2022). Impaired ability to relax pelvic floor muscles in men with chronic prostatitis/chronic pelvic pain syndrome. *Physical Therapy*, *102*(7), pzac059. https://doi.org/10.1093/ptj/pzac059

CHAPTER 7

The Bio Part 2: Passive Devices for Urinary Incontinence

As physiotherapists and prostate cancer practitioners, we are well aware of how urinary incontinence can significantly impact men's quality of life. In cases where conservative treatments fail to address the issue, or surgery may not be the best option, we may find ourselves wondering what other treatment options are available. As such, it is crucial for us to explore alternative therapies and approaches that can help our patients achieve their treatment goals and improve their overall wellbeing.

Passive devices can be a short-term or long-term solution for men with urinary incontinence, particularly for those experiencing significant symptoms or whose incontinence is impacting their emotional and mental wellbeing, as well as their ability to participate in the community. This chapter provides an overview of the two types of passive devices available and includes a discussion of a short-term clamp protocol developed by Dr. Jo Milios for use post-prostatectomy, as well as information and study results of a new male urethral insert.

PASSIVE DEVICE TYPES

Passive devices for male urinary incontinence serve two purposes: they either compress the penile urethra from the outside (clamps) or block urine passage from the inside of the urethra (such as with Contino®). These devices differ from collection devices that drain urine into a container or bag (such as with sheath systems or body-worn urinals), as the primary function of passive devices is to prevent urine from leaking out. One advantage of wearing passive devices is that by containing urine inside the urethra, it can be accumulated in the bladder, and the sensation to urinate can be normalized, leading to improved urine flow. When men are constantly leaking, they may not feel the sensation of urination (which typically occurs when the bladder is about half full), and normalizing this sensation can greatly improve their quality of life. In this regard, the use of clamps may enhance bladder behavior.

CLAMPS

The penile clamp was first documented by Lorenz Heister in 1718[1] and it was first patented in 1929 by Joseph A. Hyaxs in New York, USA. He named his invention the urethral clip, made of two parallel horizontal wire parts and one vertical part, joined together by the bottom horizontal piece where a spring load mechanism was attached to be able to adjust and be operated with a single hand. It was an adaptable urethral external compression device made of two movable pieces—each of the pieces was composed of a single length of wire.[2]

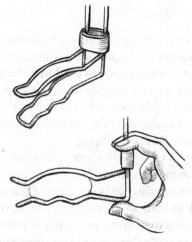

FIGURE 7.1: JOSEPH A. HYAXS URETHRAL CLIP MODEL[3]

Clamp designs have continued to improve with the intention of providing sufficient closure of the urethra without impeding circulation. They are made of materials that are compact, non-irritating, easy to wash, and capable of fitting a variety of penis sizes.[4] Most clamps today are made of stainless steel and have a plastic outer surface with rubber or silicone on the inside. They are hinged on one side to provide adjustable tension. It is recommended to avoid wearing them for long periods of time and to remove them every 3–4 hours, for instance,[5] and to change the position of the clamp slightly on the penis (for example, 1 cm above or below initial position). It was noted that distal blood flow velocity of the penis can be compromised while using the clamp with enough compression to maintain dryness (Cunningham clamp).[6]

---

1   (Schultheiss *et al.*, 2000)
2   (Hyams, 1929)
3   United State Patent Office, filed March 8, 1929. Serial No. 345,380.
4   (Edwards, 1965)
5   (Kalra *et al.*, 2015)
6   (Moore *et al.*, 2004)

Other complications that were reported, especially with long-term users were pain, urethral erosion, obstruction, and edema.[7]

Table 7.1: Most common clamp models

Brand	Picture	Information
Wiesner Incontinence Penile Clamp		• 3 sizes in one • Adjustable: 4 different pressure levels • Inside made of soft foam silicone www.wiesnerhealth.com
Bard Cunnigham Clamp		• 3 sizes (juvenile, regular, and large) • Adjustable: 5 settings • Stainless steel on the outside and foam on the inside • The manufacturer suggests having 2–3 units in hand and rotating them throughout the day to let the foam shape go back to normal. They also suggest repositioning the clamp every 2 hours[8] Bard Medical: www.bd.com
Pacey Cuff Male Incontinence Device		• 4 sizes (SM, M, L, XL) • Adjusts using Velcro • Manufacturer claims that it can be worn all day as it has circulation protection and it acts differently than a clamp https://paceycuff.com
Dribblestop Incontinence Penile Clamp		• Comes in a set of 2 • Adjustable • Inside made of hypoallergenic foam https://dribblestop.com

A study comparing Amazon reviews of penile clamps found that the majority of the reviews were positive, with most of them relating to effective incontinence control. The study identified the Wiesner and Cunningham clamps as

---

7   (Kalra *et al.*, 2015)
8   (*Bard Cunningham Penile Clamp for Male Incontinence*, n.d.)

having the most positive reviews, while the Dribblestop and Pacey Cuff had the most negative reviews. Positive reviews were mostly related to improved urinary control, while negative reviews were related to issues such as discomfort, bad design, or material. The Pacey Cuff was the most expensive among the four clamps, with a price difference of around $40. The Wiesner was the most frequently reviewed of all the penile clamps, accounting for approximately 70 percent of the reviews. [9]

Clamps used during treatment

The use of clamps during radiation therapy was demonstrated to improve bladder filling on prostate cancer patients with UI or overactive bladder. Proper bladder filling is required to displace the small bowel out of the field and to reduce the volume of bladder treated, minimizing toxicity to the tissues. Mean bladder volume in this small trial improved from 99 ml to 327 ml with the clamp.[10]

Clamp protocol by Dr. Milios, PhD (unpublished data)

This protocol was developed by physiotherapist Dr. Milios, PhD, in Australia. She has reported implementing it with over 500 patients following prostatectomy. The protocol is recommended for men experiencing severe urinary incontinence post-surgery, requiring multiple pads throughout the day, facing difficulties with proper urination due to continuous leaking of urine, or struggling with urinary incontinence and pad usage. Typically, Milios suggests initiating the protocol from four weeks post-op, but only once a urine test (to rule out a UTI) has been completed. Dr. Milios also recommends that pelvic floor exercises should be performed while utilizing a clamp, and emphasizes the importance of consistent continuation.

1. Initiate the practice of wearing the penile clamp during daytime hours, ensuring a minimum duration of two hours before emptying the bladder.
2. Keep the penile clamp on throughout the day, including during exercise, but refrain from wearing it at night.
3. Gradually extend the duration of wearing the penile clamp to two to three hours initially, progressing to four hours, while being cautious not to wear it if experiencing any pain or discomfort.
4. Allocate one day each week without wearing the penile clamp to allow the skin to rest and to assess bladder functionality (refer to details in Table 7.2).
5. Evaluate progress after four weeks, considering the possibility of

9   (Lee *et al.*, 2021)
10 (Malone *et al.*, 2015)

reducing or discontinuing the use of clamps if experiencing dryness or requiring fewer than three pads per day.

6. It is crucial to note that the penile clamp should never be used as a long-term solution; it is intended solely as a temporary aid for specific occasions or during highly strenuous exercises.

Table 7.2: Dr. Milios' clamp protocol

Clamp recommendation	Wiesner Penile Clamp
Duration	6 days a week for a maximum of 6 weeks
24-hour pad test Day 1 (Week 1–6)	NO CLAMP USAGE Measure the weight of pads used over a 24-hour period using a kitchen scale. Weight = total weight – (weight of dry pad × number of pads used) Repeat this measurement once a week for 5 weeks.
Protocol Day 2–7 (Week 1–6)	CLAMP USAGE Wear the clamp during the day (excluding night-time), removing it every 2–4 hours to urinate. After removal, reposition the clamp slightly (e.g., 1 cm above or below its previous position). Repeat this process for 4–6 weeks, 6 times a week.

Please note that this protocol is based on unpublished data from Dr. Jo Milios, PhD, and should be implemented under professional supervision.

URETHRAL INSERT: CONTINO®

The Contino® device is a Canadian product that has completed a five-year product evaluation study and is currently undergoing a post-market clinical follow up study as required for expanding its international licencing. The Contino® device was found to decrease urine loss and enhance patient perception of urinary incontinence with minimal adverse effects, indicating it as a feasible non-invasive alternative for men experiencing SUI.[11] This Canadian licenced urethral insert device, classified as a class 2 medical device, requires a clinician (such as physiotherapists, medical doctors, or registered nurses) for fitting and prescribing. It can serve as another conservative management option for those with moderate to severe urinary incontinence caused mainly by sphincteric deficiency (passive or active urinary incontinence not associated with urgency). Life 360 Innovations, the company behind Contino®, provides patients with support, screening, and referral to clinics that are

---

11   (Cuaj, 2020)

trained to fit the device. They also offer training to clinicians who meet the qualification criteria for fitting.

Interview with Bob Orr, president, co-founder, and CEO of Life 160 Innovations

How did you get involved with Contino®?

A friend of a family, who was an aircraft engineer and was struggling with urinary incontinence after radical prostatectomy surgery, approached me with this idea of an urethral plug that he has developed and created over the past three years. He had been using the device on himself and it was effectively keeping him dry and normalizing his urinary function. In 2010, myself, my father, and this friend incorporated the company, and for the past five years the product was re-engineered by a recognized medical device prototyping department of the British Columbia Institute of Technology, patented and developed into a more commercialized product. In 2015, the product was commercialized and submitted into an investigational preliminary study to test the efficacy and safety of the device in improving urinary incontinence. The study helped us to further improve the technology by creating 16 different sizes. The abstract of this foundational study was published in 2020, showing reduction in urine loss with minor adverse events.[12] The adverse events found in the clinical trial were very mild bleeding and mild discomfort resolved without any further medical intervention.

Can you briefly explain the design, material, and function of this urethral device?

The design required approximately 10,000 hours of engineering refinement, manufacture validation, and verification. The device is 4.5 inches long, with standardizer lanyard and tab, with different head sizes. The head size diameter uses a French catheter system as it is a well-known system for the medical community. The system includes the device and a clear, hard, plastic inserting tool. The Contino® is made of a very high-quality plastic manufactured in Germany with bio-compatibility requirements, used usually in permanent implantable devices, which has satisfied ISO10993 standards. It has a very simple design to make it easily reproduced and safe for patients. Usually, it is designed to sit inside the penile urethra in the transition space between the penile urethra and the glans, but it can vary by people. Usually, the device can be accommodated well in the penile urethra as it is highly distensible, contrary to the glans urethra. The device stays in place due to the combination of the

---

12   (Cuaj, 2020)

shape of the device, the placement, the material, the surface finishing, the urethral resting tone, and by being properly managed by the user. The users are recommended to go through a bladder diary routine to recognize their habits and to train themselves to have regular urination intervals. It is recommended for them to urinate every 2–3 hours depending on their fluid intake, as the device is intentionally designed to pop out with a large increase in pressure.

What are the advantages you see with Contino® compared to other passive devices such as clamps?

Compared to our product, clamps are relatively cheap products not intended to be worn 24/7, and I am not sure if the medical community fully supports them, as adverse events can be great. We have heard anecdotally that people who have been users of clamps before they come to our product have developed strictures and can have more challenges using or inserting our product. Clamps can be very effective on a temporary basis, for example, during exercises. On the other hand, the Contino® device can be used very effectively during exercises, but also on a daily basis for those who have passive incontinence. The Contino is designed for long-term use, and has much fewer risks compared to clamps and surgical procedures.

Any challenges or limitations that you have encountered?

Some patients want quick solutions for their urinary problems, but sometimes their urinary concerns may not be as straightforward. Some patients quit before they give the product a chance as it may take them 2–3 weeks to get used to the device. We realized that, for the product to work effectively, a system was needed to be put in place. We offer consultations before they are scheduled to see a professional fitter, to screen and coach them about our product, and also teach them about their own urinary habits and concerns. To avoid urethral irritation or sensitivity, we also developed a protocol of slowly progressing them to the size they were fitted for, with step-by-step instructions on how to progress them in subsequent weeks. We have introduced "The Get Started Guide" and a system of professional follow-ups, helping users adhere to the product in the most effective way. It is a combination of the system put in place and the Contino® for it to work successfully.

Do you think there are any risks for this device to progressively dilate the urethra?

There might be. Our inventor, who has been the user for the longest time (over ten years) noticed that he had to go up one or two sizes. He is over 90 years old, and he feels his tissue is also not as pliable as before, and maybe that is why he had to go up in size. We also noticed that the device may be self-regulating in a way, for example, it won't fit or distend a smaller urethra, even in certain users who push themselves to their limit by wanting to be dry at any cost. We have observed, in a very few cases, patients who may have lost their urethral pliability (or tone) after too many urethral procedures, and who had to go up in sizes for the device to stay in.

What are your strategic plans/goals for Contino®? Do you have an idea when this product would be available in other countries?

We have patents in 20 different countries, and are currently conducting a post-market clinical trial to be able to compete with the international market. We are also looking to develop a female version of the product, and possibly a fecal device. We additionally manufactured a strap that goes around the penis to help keep the device in place during more strenuous activities.

Any other comment?

We believe that the Contino® not only can help decrease urinary leakages in men, but can also maybe be used as a bladder treatment, as we have been noticing increased bladder responses, for example: increased bladder capacity and sensitization, increased urge reflex, improved urination stream, and decreased post-void residual volume. We hope to in the future present more quantifiable data to support these hypotheses.

CASE STUDY

In June 2016, a healthy and active 70-year-old man was diagnosed with prostate cancer and an aggressive tumor in the pelvic region during a transurethral resection of the prostate (TURP). More cancer was later discovered in his bladder and successfully removed with no recurrence. The patient underwent radiation treatment for the PC and pelvic tumor, which was effective in reducing the pelvic tumor and did not result in urinary incontinence post-treatment.

In April 2019, the patient underwent a successful hemipelvectomy to remove the pelvic tumor, but partial removal of the pelvic and pubic bones was necessary, and a repair was required to the bladder neck and internal urethral sphincter region. Following the surgery, the patient experienced stress urinary incontinence (SUI), urinary retention, post-void residual urine, and urinary tract infections (UTI). While in the hospital, a condom catheter was used to manage his SUI partially. All symptoms except for the SUI had resolved before discharge. However, after discharge, his SUI worsened, requiring four or more adult briefs per day, and he experienced increased frequency of voiding at night and decreased urine volume. A follow-up cystoscopy with his urologist five months later revealed nothing significant.

The patient reported a reduction in physical activity, social activities, and sleep quality, which had deteriorated completely. Due to radiation treatments, the patient was ineligible for another invasive surgical operation to treat his SUI. Frustrated with inadequate symptom management and non-surgical options, he was referred to Contino® by a healthcare professional. In February 2020, he attended an appointment with a pelvic floor physiotherapist who fits Contino®, but due to a meatal stricture, the Contino® sizing gauge could not be inserted. His baseline score on the validated International Consultation on Incontinence Questionnaire (ICIQ) scale was 9. His urologist completed a cystoscopy and found nothing significant.

At a second appointment eight months later, size 28 of the Contino® device was successfully inserted and removed by the nurse liaison. However, the patient experienced some difficulties and minor bleeding when he reattempted at home. Consequently, he was provided with a range of smaller sizes, allowing him to gradually onboard the Contino®. Another cystoscopy with his urologist in January 2021 revealed nothing significant. The patient discussed his usage of the Contino® device, and the urologist had no objections to continued usage. By March 2021, the patient was back to using size 28, demonstrating successful device application. He had eliminated the use of adult briefs and switched to pads, with an estimated 50 percent urine loss reduction. Over time with continued individualized support and consultation from the nurse liaison, he increased to size 32 of the Contino®. They also identified optimal personalized placement of the device that best suited his anatomy.

Since using the Contino® device, the patient's urine leakage has reduced by 100 percent according to his subjective assessment, and he has not had any adverse events requiring medical intervention since 2020. His ICIQ assessment decreased to a score of 2, indicating meaningful improvements as interpreted by the FDA. He now reports no pain, discomfort, or leakage with the Contino®, as well as significant improvements in his sleep hygiene and quality of life.

CONCLUSION

This chapter discussed the use of passive devices, including clamps and Contino®, as a potential option for men experiencing urinary incontinence due to urethral insufficiency. These devices can be considered when other conservative treatment options, such as pelvic floor rehabilitation, have not been effective, and when patients are seeking an alternative to pads or surgery. Passive devices have shown promise in reducing urinary leakages, improving bladder filling, and normalizing bladder sensations and function, which can ultimately improve quality of life and social participation for prostate cancer survivors. However, it's important to note that these devices may not be suitable for everyone, and patient-centered care is crucial in considering individual goals and cultural perspectives when discussing treatment options.

REFERENCES

Bard Cunningham Penile Clamp for Male Incontinence (n.d.). Retrieved January 30, 2023, from www.vitalitymedical.com/bard-adjustable-cunningham-clamp.html

Cuaj, E. (2020). CUA 2020 Annual Meeting Abstracts. Canadian Urological Association Journal, 14(6S2), Article 6S2. https://doi.org/10.5489/cuaj.6732

Edwards, L.E. (1965). An easily operated incontinence clamp. British Medical Journal, 2(5468), 985.

Hyams, J.A. (1929). A new penis clip. Journal of Urology, 22(1), 121–124. https://doi.org/10.1016/S0022-5347(17)73018-2

Kalra, S., Srinivas, P.R., Manikandan, R., & Dorairajan, L.N. (2015). Urethral diverticulum: A potential hazard of penile clamp application for male urinary incontinence. BMJ Case Reports, 2015, bcr2015209957. https://doi.org/10.1136/bcr-2015-209957

Lee, A., Mmonu, N.A., Thomas, H., Rios, N., Enriquez, A., & Breyer, B.N. (2021). Qualitative analysis of Amazon customer reviews of penile clamps for male urinary incontinence. Neurourology and Urodynamics, 40(1), 384–390. https://doi.org/10.1002/nau.24572

Malone, S., Wright, G., Lacelle, M., Buckley, L., et al. (2015). Evaluation of a penile clamp to improve bladder filling in patients undergoing radiation therapy for prostate cancer. International Journal of Radiation Oncology, Biology, Physics, 93(3), E210–E211. https://doi.org/10.1016/j.ijrobp.2015.07.1082

Moore, K.N., Schieman, S., Ackerman, T., Dzus, H.Y., Metcalfe, J.B., & Voaklander, D.C. (2004). Assessing comfort, safety, and patient satisfaction with three commonly used penile compression devices. Urology, 63(1), 150–154. https://doi.org/10.1016/j.urology.2003.08.034

Schultheiss, D., Höfner, K., Oelke, M., Grünewald, V., & Jonas, U. (2000). Historical aspects of the treatment of urinary incontinence. European Urology, 38(3), 352–362. https://doi.org/10.1159/000020306

CHAPTER 8

Exercise and Prostate Cancer

Is exercise safe during and after prostate cancer treatments?

Furthermore, can exercise interfere with delivery of treatment or recovery after treatment, or is it associated with the risk of cancer recurrence and progression?

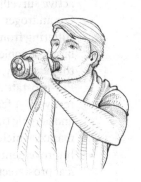

More specifically, what kind of exercise would be beneficial to prostate cancer survivors (PCS)?

This chapter's intent is to answer these common questions and to highlight studies and data regarding the effect of exercise in prostate cancer survivors' function, activities, and psychosocial outcomes.

A REVIEW OF THE LITERATURE

According to recent studies, exercise seems to be probably the most effective way to improve a variety of cancer patients' quality of life, cardiovascular health, mood, fatigue, treatment response (including chemotherapy[1]), anxiety, depression, and pain.[2, 3, 4] Moreover, exercise can improve cancer treatment completion, reduce anxiety pre-treatment, and may improve cancer recurrence and survival in prostate cancer survivors.[5] Exercise has also been suggested to alleviate chemotherapy induced peripheral neuropathy through molecular, cellular, and neural mechanisms, by improving mitochondrial function, reducing axonal degeneration, and reducing inflammation.[6] Additionally, pre-rehabilitation can potentially facilitate post-prostatectomy surgical recovery by improving physical reserve capacity, especially for those who have poor physical and muscle performance prior to surgery.[7]

1   (Yang et al., 2021)
2   (Seguin & Nelson, 2003)
3   (Carrasco et al., 2020)
4   (Wollesen et al., 2017)
5   (Kang et al., 2021)
6   (Chung et al., 2022)
7   (Singh et al., 2017)

Below are some important research highlights:

- A 2022 study demonstrated that a 12-week high intensity interval training program (HIIT) significantly improved total prostate cancer-specific anxiety, hormonal symptoms, perceived stress, and self-esteem in prostate cancer patients on active surveillance.[8]
- A HIIT program can also improve cardiovascular function, and reduce PSA levels and growth of prostate cancer cell line, without increasing testosterone levels in men who have localized prostate cancer under active surveillance.[9]
- For androgen deprivation therapy (ADT) patients, who are generally suffering from testosterone withdrawal, a six-month program combining aerobics and strength training helped to improve cardiorespiratory capacity, resting fat oxidation, glucose, and body composition.[10]
- Pre-prostatectomy exercise training may benefit patients' surgical recovery. A feasibility study demonstrated that a six-week resistance and aerobic training can aid in improving physical and muscle performance, which were maintained at six weeks post-surgery.[11]
- Improvements in quality of life were also seen in robotic-assisted radical prostatectomy patients after six months' home based resistance training intervention.[12]
- An exercise program of 2–3 days per week, including impact loading, and 20–40 minutes' moderate to high intensity (60–85% of maximal heart rate (HRmax)) resistance training focusing on major upper and lower body muscle groups, showed a reduction in pain in androgen deprivation therapy (ADT) and pelvic radiation therapy patients.[13]
- It was suggested that exercise may prevent or treat chemotherapy induced peripheral neuropathy (CIPN) through effects in the peripheral and central nervous system, as well through psychosocial mechanisms. Exercise has been shown to enhance protein production responsible for the survival and maintenance of neurons; have anti-inflammatory effects; potentialize mitochondrial function; protect against axonal degeneration; and to have an effect on psychosocial components that will influence pain perception, such as mood, depression, anxiety, fatigue, self-efficacy, and benefit expectation.[14]
- Vigorous activities (quantified as a metabolic equivalent of task (MET) >6), such as jogging, running, bicycling, lap swimming, tennis, squash/

---

8   (Kang *et al.*, 2022)
9   (Kang *et al.*, 2021)
10 (Wall *et al.*, 2017)
11 (Singh *et al.*, 2017)
12 (Ashton *et al.*, 2021)
13 (Schumacher *et al.*, 2021)
14 (Chung *et al.*, 2022)

racquetball, and stair climbing, practicing on average 4–6 hours a week, can contribute to 30% lower risk of advanced prostate cancer and 25% lower risk of lethal prostate cancer. See Table 8.1 for examples of various activities' MET values.[15]

- Resistance training can significantly improve upper and lower limb muscle strength in men aged 60–90 years. Intensity, training periods, and total time under tension were variables with greatest effects on muscle strength.[16] The benefits of resistance training extend beyond muscle strength and hypertrophy, but it is essential to improve functional activities, posture, and balance, and to reduce the risk of falls and hospitalization.[17, 18, 19] In terms of method of training, power training (moving the weight faster in the lifting phase) may have an increase in physical function compared to traditional weight training in healthy older adults.[20]

- Men with metastatic bone disease may also benefit from a carefully designed exercise program. A pilot study suggested that a 12-week, 60-minutes, twice-a-week resistance training exercise program, which was carefully monitored and designed to minimize mechanical force on affected bone cancer area, can be safe and improve physical function, physical activity, and lean mass in this population.[21]

- Lastly, physical activity does not seem to be associated with increasing risk of prostate cancer, and it seems to be safe during oncological treatment.[22]

Table 8.1: MET values for physical activities

Information retrieved from The Compendium of Physical Activities Tracking Guide.[23]

Activity	MET value
Light activities	*>3*
Sitting at rest, sleeping	1
Watching TV	1.3
Sexual activity, moderate effort	1.8
Standing	2

cont.

15 (Pernar *et al.*, 2019)
16 (Borde *et al.*, 2015)
17 (Seguin & Nelson, 2003)
18 (Carrasco *et al.*, 2020)
19 (Wollesen *et al.*, 2017)
20 (Balachandran *et al.*, 2022)
21 (Cormie *et al.*, 2013)
22 (Pernar *et al.*, 2019)
23 (Ainsworth *et al.*, n.d.)

Activity	MET value
Boat fishing	2
Grocery shopping	2.3
Light house chores	2.5
Hatha yoga	2.5
Moderate activities	*3–6*
Pilates	3
Cleaning, mopping, moderate effort	3.5
Building a fence	3.8
Power yoga	4
Leisure bicycling	4
Circuit training, moderate effort	4.3
Spreading dirt with a shovel	5
Elliptical trainer, moderate effort	5
Snow shoveling, by hand, moderate effort	5.3
Water aerobics	5.3
Ballroom dancing (fast)	5.5
Vigorous activities	*>6*
Roofing	6
Aerobic high impact	7.3
Rowing, stationary, 100 watts, moderate effort	7
Jogging	7
Skiing, general	7
Squash	7.3
Bicycling, stationary, general	7.5
Running, 6 mph (10 min/mile)	9.8
Swimming laps, freestyle, fast, vigorous effort	9.8
Rope skipping	12.3
Bicycling, mountain, uphill, vigorous	14

RECOMMENDATIONS

The American Cancer Society's Nutrition and Physical Activity Guidelines for Cancer Survivors and the WHO (World Health Organization) recommend a minimum of 150 minutes of moderate or 75 minutes of vigorous aerobic exercise per week.[24] Exercises should be tailored to each individual's abilities and medical history. Resistance 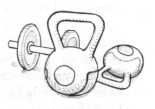 training is also recommended at least twice a week, and is of great benefit in the older adult population.[25]

Supervised exercise programs by a therapist or physiologist can be of more benefit than home programs or non-supervised exercise programs.[26] The US Department of Health and Human Services (HHS) also suggests that adding balance training into older adults' exercise programs can be beneficial to improve functional abilities.[27] A flexibility and stretching program is recommended to maintain joint mobility and help enable older adults to continue to perform functional tasks, as declining flexibility can significantly impair an individual's ability to accomplish daily activities and perform exercise.[28] There aren't any standardized parameters for stretching protocols; however, a 10-week, 40-minute, 3-days-a-week, major lower extremity muscle-group stretching program helped to improve flexibility, range of motion, and exercise performance—improving knee extension strength, knee extension, and flexion endurance and jumping performance.[29] A recent study suggested that a 30-second hamstring stretch is probably the preferred duration to optimally increase knee range of motion and minimize strain on the nerve roots and central nervous system.[30] Most exercise study protocols recommend having a warm-up of at least 5 minutes and cool down sessions of at least 10 minutes.

Yoga and tai-qi, which have been shown to be beneficial to improve the quality of life of cancer patients, can be an alternate mode of exercise for strength, balance, and flexibility training.[31] For those prostate cancer survivors who are deconditioned, or immediately post-op, multiple shorter bouts of 5–10 minutes (to accumulate at least 20 minutes per day) is recommended, progressing to longer sessions of 20 minutes during most days of the week.[32]

According to Joy Egilson (Zoom interview, May 17, 2022), certified athletic therapist and a clinical exercise physiologist who is involved in

---

24 (Rock *et al.*, 2012)
25 (Seguin & Nelson, 2003)
26 (Baumann *et al.*, 2012)
27 (*2018 Physical Activity Guidelines Advisory Committee Scientific Report*, n.d.)
28 (Pollock *et al.*, 1998)
29 (Kokkonen *et al.*, 2007)
30 (Moustafa *et al.*, 2021)
31 (Danhauer *et al.*, 2017)
32 (Jones *et al.*, 2010)

community-based and research exercise programs for prostate cancer survivors (including a research program for men with bone metastasis), it is important to identify first each individual's starting point before prescribing an exercise program. Joy suggested that for many people who never exercised before or are very sedentary, introducing movement and reducing sedentary times can be a way to start. She believes that home-based functional exercises can be as impactful for some men as a structured exercise program. She says that the key to success with this population is to build a program that would be "fail-proof," for example, starting out with exercise suggestions which will easily fit into their routine, like adding 4–5 sit-to-stands after they get up from a chair and a wall push-up after they brush their teeth. More specifically, Joy usually starts with postural and core control and then moves towards the "big" movements such as hinging, squatting, and lifting, which are essential movements for day-to-day activities. Joy also believes that deconstructing the meaning of exercising can help people become more engaged—for instance, educating prostate cancer survivors in all the different ways one can exercise.

Jo Milios, PhD, (Zoom interview, June 7, 2022), registered physiotherapist and founder of PROST! Inc. (a non-profit exercise program for prostate cancer survivors), found that when you incorporate an evidence-based exercise group program in a space which will be attractive to males, such as the local football club, can help improve general interest and adherence. She also suggested that providing prostate cancer survivors with a light-hearted supportive environment for them to meet and exercise together can have a profound effect on their physical health and mental status, and can transform lives. Dr. Milios recommends incorporating pelvic floor muscle training within the strength training program, as well as outdoor cardio activities, pilates, and yoga. The PROST! manuals (see Resources at end of chapter) can be purchased to help clinicians and support leaders set up the exercise program in any practice or gymnasium facility.

Outlined here are some of Joy Egilson's exercise suggestions for the older population:

- Inchworm—help to build strategies to get up from the floor
- Wall push-ups (triceps strengthening)—help with bed mobility and get-up from a chair
- Bird Dog—core connection and activation

EXERCISE 8.1: INCHWORM

1) Inchworm, starting position	2) Inchworm, descend	3) Inchworm, hand-walking
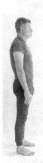	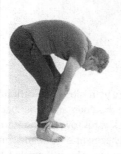	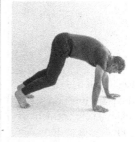
To begin this exercise, stand tall at the back of your mat with your feet hip-width apart. Take a deep breath in and, as you exhale, feel a gentle connection with the ground beneath you. Activate your deeper abdominal muscles by drawing your belly button towards your spine. This will help you to stabilize your core and maintain good posture throughout your practice.	Maintain the gentle activation of your abdominal muscles as you slowly roll down through your spine, bending your knees and allowing your hands to reach towards the ground. Keep your weight evenly distributed between your feet and avoid locking your knees, to protect your joints.	While continuing to engage your deep abdominal muscles, walk your hands towards the top of your mat, keeping your spine aligned and your neck long. To maintain proper alignment, gaze slightly forward of your hands rather than looking down. This will help you avoid straining your neck and keep your focus on your practice.

4) Inchworm, plank position	5) Inchworm, moving to the back of the mat
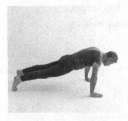	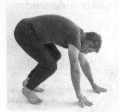 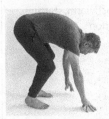
When you have reached the plank position, maintain engagement of your deeper abdominal muscles by keeping your rib cage connected to your spine and gently pulling your belly button towards your spine. Breathe in and out through your nose, focusing on keeping your breath smooth and steady. Remember to keep your body in a straight line from head to heels, avoiding any sagging or arching in your lower back.	Hike your hips back without collapsing through the shoulders and lower back. While hand-walking backwards towards the starting position, maintain engagement of your abdominal muscles to protect your lower back. If needed, bend your knees to help keep your spine straight. Once you have returned to the starting position, roll up to standing, one vertebra at a time, keeping your neck relaxed and your shoulders down. From here, you can begin the sequence again.

Repetitions of this exercise may vary between individuals depending on their level of experience and fitness. For beginners, it's important to focus on rolling down through the spine and shifting your weight onto your hands without overstretching or overworking your muscles. Avoid walking your hands too far forward as this may compromise your form and lead to strain in your shoulders or wrists.

EXERCISE 8.2: WALL PUSH-UPS

To perform wall push-ups, stand tall in front of a wall with your arms straight and your hands touching the wall at shoulder height. Your elbows should be bent at a 90-degree angle, with your wrists aligned to your shoulders. For triceps push-ups, keep your elbows close to your body as you bring your body towards the wall. Maintain proper alignment by keeping your spine and neck tall and facing forward, and engage your shoulder blades by pulling them down and towards each other. For wider-grip push-ups, move your hands outside of shoulder-width instead of directly below your shoulders, keeping the shoulders and elbows at a 90-degree angle. This will target your chest and shoulder muscles. Remember to breathe throughout the exercise and adjust the intensity as needed by adjusting the distance between your body and the wall.

Repetitions of this exercise may vary between individuals depending on their level of experience and fitness. The goal of the exercise is to challenge your muscles and create fatigue, so it's normal to experience some shaking or trembling. However, if you feel pain or discomfort, it's important to adjust the intensity or seek guidance from a fitness professional.

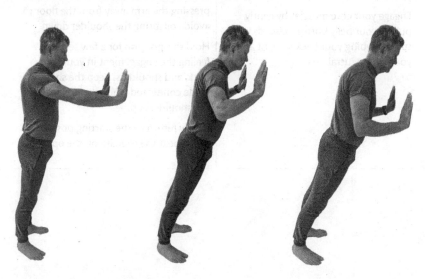

EXERCISE 8.3: BIRD DOG

The Bird Dog is a bodyweight exercise that targets your core, back, and gluteal muscles. Here are the steps to perform a Bird Dog:

1) Starting position	2) Arm variation
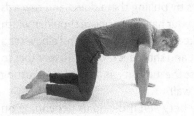	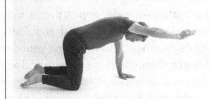
Start on your hands and knees, with your hands directly under your shoulders and your knees directly under your hips. Engage your core muscles by gently pulling your belly button towards your spine, keeping your back straight and your neck neutral.	While keeping your hips and shoulders leveled and avoiding any twisting or tilting in your body, extend your right arm straight out in front of you. Keep pressing the arm away from the floor to avoid collapsing the shoulder down. Hold this position for a few seconds, feeling the engagement in your core, back, and shoulders. Keep the shoulder blade connected while avoiding hiking the shoulders up. Slowly return to the starting position and repeat the exercise on the opposite side

3) Leg variation

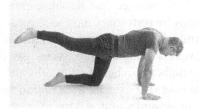

This is a progression from the arm variation. While keeping your hips and shoulders leveled and avoiding any twisting or tilting in your body, shift your weight slightly forward to extend your right leg, keeping the hip bones facing down towards the mat. Try to avoid rotating the hips out.

Hold this position for a few seconds, feeling the engagement in your core, back, and glute muscles.

Slowly return to the starting position and repeat the exercise on the opposite side

4) Full version

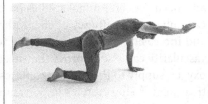

Once you are able to perform arm and leg variations you are ready to try the full Bird Dog version.

While keeping your hips and shoulders leveled and avoiding any twisting or tilting in your body, extend your right arm straight out in front of you while simultaneously extending your left leg straight back behind you.

Hold this position for a few seconds, feeling the engagement in your core, back, and glute muscles.

Slowly return to the starting position and repeat the exercise on the opposite side, extending your left arm and right leg.

Tips

- Make sure to keep your movements slow and controlled, avoiding any jerking or bouncing motions.
- Focus on maintaining a straight line from your head to your heels throughout the exercise.
- Perform 8–10 repetitions on each side, gradually increasing the number of repetitions as your strength and stability improve.

EXERCISING WITH ADVANCED PROSTATE CANCER

Exercise therapy has shown promise in improving outcomes for patients with advanced cancer. Animal studies have demonstrated that aerobic exercise can enhance the efficacy of chemotherapy by restoring tumor vasculature and increasing blood supply to the tumor.[33, 34, 35] This increase in tumor vascularity can also improve the effectiveness of radiotherapy, as increased oxygen supply to the tumor promotes a higher number of cell deaths after treatment.[36] However, it's important to note that exercise prescription for this population needs to be carefully planned and monitored to ensure it is well-tolerated, safe, and effective. Patients with advanced prostate cancer may present with complex clinical issues that require a tailored exercise program to minimize potential risks and maximize benefits. For instance, patients with bone metastases may need to avoid high-impact load into the metastases sites to prevent fractures, while patients with neuropathy may need to avoid exercises that exacerbate symptoms. Therefore, exercise programs for advanced prostate cancer patients should be designed and implemented by trained professionals, such as exercise physiologists or physical therapists, with experience working with cancer patients.

EXERCISE THERAPY FOR CARDIOTOXICITY IN CANCER PATIENTS

Zoth and colleagues suggested that oncology exercise therapy could be used as diagnosis, prevention, and treatment of cardiovascular complications (cardiotoxicity) resulting from cancer treatments, and that it should ideally be prescribed immediately after diagnoses.[37] The "Proposed Decision Support Algorithm for Cardio-Oncology and Cardiac Rehabilitation" (CORE) recommended performing screening and cardiac monitoring—for example by regular monitoring VO2peak—during cancer therapy. These screening tools could be used to determine which patients should be surveyed and receive specialized exercise therapy or be referred to community exercise programs.[38] Although the *degree* of cardiovascular events after prostate cancer treatments, such as androgen deprivation therapy (ADT), radiation therapy, and chemotherapy drugs (such as Docetaxel), are still inconclusive, aerobic exercises that are properly monitored may be advantageous in improving cardiovascular status of prostate cancer patients by preventing cardiac cell

---

33   (Schadler *et al.*, 2016)
34   (Betof *et al.*, 2015)
35   (Betof *et al.*, 2013)
36   (Jordan & Sonveaux, 2012)
37   (Zoth *et al.*, 2023)
38   (Bonsignore *et al.*, 2021)

damage, and reducing oxidative stress.[39] The "ABCDE" framework proposed by Bhatia and colleagues includes exercise (E) as essential to minimize risk of cardiac events in prostate cancer patients.[40]

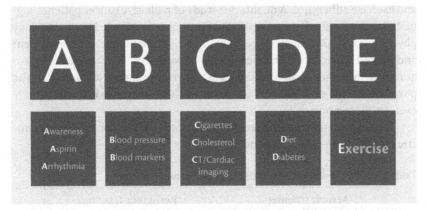

FIGURE 8.1: THE "ABCDE" ALGORITHM FOR MANAGING CARDIOVASCULAR RISK FACTORS FOR PROSTATE CANCER SURVIVORS[41]

EXERCISE ENGAGEMENT

Although this chapter calls attention to many biopsychosocial health benefits of exercise therapy in prostate cancer care, there may be an increased need for supporting prostate cancer patients with physical activity behavior change, as the majority may not participate or engage in activities reaching the amount recommended by the health organizations. Prevalence rates for prostate cancer survivors engaging in the recommended amount of aerobic exercises may be around 40 percent and although not reported, it is suspected that rates may even be lower in meeting resistance training guidelines.[42] Contrasting to these high rates of reduced physical activity participation, the majority of PCS receiving ADT treatments seem to express the acceptance of or willingness to engage in fitness programs,[43] showing a gap in their supportive care for facilitating PCS in enhancing exercise participation. Some barriers noted by prostate cancer physicians and clinicians in promoting physical activity were lack of consultation time and lack of confidence in providing information about physical activity[44], highlighting the importance

---

39   (Zoth *et al.*, 2023)
40   (Bhatia *et al.*, 2016)
41   (Based on Campbell *et al.,* 2020)
42   (Cormie *et al.*, 2015)
43   (Harrington *et al.*, 2013)
44   (Fox *et al.*, 2019)

for improving the education on physical activity promotion and care plan coordination among oncology clinicians.

Group exercise programs led by qualified health professionals, such as physiotherapists, may help increase prostate cancer survivors' motivation and exercise adherence. A qualitative study of palliative cancer patients suggested that an outpatient group-format exercise program led by an oncology physiotherapist (in a hospital setting) improved their exercise commitment and helped to increase their perception of wellness.[45] Group exercise programs for prostate cancer survivors set in environments attractive to the population—for example the local football club—may also help to improve exercise motivation.

Table 8.2 summarizes the recommendations of clinical exercising parameters for prostate cancer patients[46]

Table 8.2: PCS clinical exercise parameter recommendations

	Aerobic training	Resistance training
Goals	Improve physical fitness, QoL Improve body composition Decrease pain Reduce fatigue Decrease anxiety, stress Decrease PSA Decrease risk of advanced PC Anti-inflammatory effects	Improve physical fitness, QoL Improve body composition Improve balance Decrease pain Reduce fatigue Decrease anxiety, stress Decrease PSA Decrease risk of falls Anti-inflammatory effects
Start	Pre-op During radiation, chemotherapy, ADT, and active surveillance 48 h post-op: low intensities 6 weeks post-op: intensive and extensive if possible	Pre-op During radiation, chemotherapy, ADT, and active surveillance 48 h to 6–8 weeks post-op: low intensities
	During radiation and ADT	During radiation and ADT
	48 h post-op: low intensities	48 h post-op: low intensities
	6 weeks post-op: intensive and extensive if possible	6 weeks post-op: intensive and extensive if possible

45 (Paltiel *et al.*, 2009)
46 (Baumann *et al.*, 2012)

Duration	Long-term	Long-term
		At least 12 weeks to change muscle composition
Sessions	2–3 sessions per week 75 minutes of vigorous or 150 minutes of moderate intensity	2–3 sessions per week for all major muscle groups
Intensity	60–80% of the HRmax	60–85% of the 1-RM
	50–75% of the VO2max Met over 6 if able	

Adapted and modified from Baumann et al., 2012.[47]
QoL: Quality of life
HRmax: Maximum heart rate
VO2max: Maximum oxygen consumption
RM: Repetition Maximum

CASE STUDY

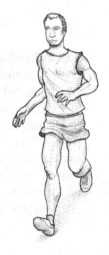

A 55-year-old client who attended one of my group pre-prostatectomy education classes came for a follow-up appointment one year after his surgery. He looked noticeably different, having lost 50 pounds and appearing physically fit and healthy. After being diagnosed with prostate cancer, he did some research on exercise and learned about the benefits of nutrition and lifestyle changes for improving his cancer outcome. He hired a personal trainer and began a weight management and fitness program. Within a year, he was very satisfied with his progress, feeling strong, leaner, and happier overall. His exercise routine consisted of running 5–6 km, 3–4 times a week, and strength training twice a week. He reported that running helped him maintain dryness (he had previously experienced urinary incontinence post-surgery) and also helped with his anxiety and depression. He was so inspired by his recovery that he became involved in community programs and meetings with the goal of sharing his experience and motivating other men after prostate cancer surgery.

---

47 (Baumann et al., 2012)

SPECIAL CONSIDERATIONS ON HERNIAS

Patients who undergo prostatectomy are at an increased risk of developing inguinal hernias, especially if they had retropubic procedures.[48] Increased intra-abdominal pressure (for example in obese individuals), weakness of the abdominal wall, wound healing complications, and abdominal surgeries are risk factors for ventral hernias.[49, 50] Although there is limited data on conservative preventive measures for ventral hernias, pre-surgical lower abdominal strengthening (core) and co-ordination exercises may be indicated for those having prostate cancer surgery. There seems to be an association between pelvic postural control (for example for those individuals with anterior pelvic tilt) and sports hernia.[51] An anterior pelvic tilt can promote weakening on the abdominal wall and shortening of hip flexors, adductors, and paraspinal muscles. Assessing cancer survivors pre-surgically and prescribing exercises which can lengthen those shortened muscles and strengthen the abdominal wall may potentially prevent the appearance or reappearance of hernias post-op.

EXERCISE SAFETY

It is recommended that medical screening and exercise safety evaluations are conducted before prescribing or referring prostate cancer survivors to an exercise program. Oncological patients may have other comorbidities or medical conditions which may impact exercise safety; therefore, a complete history and evaluation of their cardiac, pulmonary, neurological, and musculoskeletal systems should be done before they engage in physical activity. Questionnaires such as the Physical Activity Readiness Questionnaire for Everyone (PAR-Q+; see following pages) or the online questionnaire ePARmed-X+ can be used as pre-participation screening tools.[52]

---

48 (Alder *et al.*, 2020)
49 (Barranquero *et al.*, 2020)
50 (Mahfouz & Al-Juaid, 2021)
51 (Waryasz, 2010)
52 https://eparmedx.com

2023 PAR-Q+

The Physical Activity Readiness Questionnaire for Everyone

The health benefits of regular physical activity are clear; more people should engage in physical activity every day of the week. Participating in physical activity is very safe for MOST people. This questionnaire will tell you whether it is necessary for you to seek further advice from your doctor OR a qualified exercise professional before becoming more physically active.

GENERAL HEALTH QUESTIONS

Please read the 7 questions below carefully and answer each one honestly: check YES or NO.	YES	NO
1) Has your doctor ever said that you have a heart condition ☐ OR high blood pressure ☐?	☐	☐
2) Do you feel pain in your chest at rest, during your daily activities of living, OR when you do physical activity?	☐	☐
3) Do you lose balance because of dizziness OR have you lost consciousness in the last 12 months? Please answer NO if your dizziness was associated with over-breathing (including during vigorous exercise).	☐	☐
4) Have you ever been diagnosed with another chronic medical condition (other than heart disease or high blood pressure)? PLEASE LIST CONDITION(S) HERE: _____	☐	☐
5) Are you currently taking prescribed medications for a chronic medical condition? PLEASE LIST CONDITION(S) HERE: _____	☐	☐
6) Do you currently have (or have had within the past 12 months) a bone, joint, or soft tissue (muscle, ligament, or tendon) problem that could be made worse by becoming more physically active? Please answer NO if you had a problem in the past, but it does not limit your current ability to be physically active. PLEASE LIST CONDITION(S) HERE: _____	☐	☐
7) Has your doctor ever said that you should only do medically supervised physical activity?	☐	☐

☑ **If you answered NO to all of the questions above, you are cleared for physical activity. Please sign the PARTICIPANT DECLARATION. You do not need to complete Pages 2 and 3.**
- ► Start becoming much more physically active - start slowly and build up gradually.
- ► Follow Global Physical Activity Guidelines for your age (https://www.who.int/publications/i/item/9789240015128).
- ► You may take part in a health and fitness appraisal.
- ► If you are over the age of 45 yr and NOT accustomed to regular vigorous to maximal effort exercise, consult a qualified exercise professional before engaging in this intensity of exercise.
- ► If you have any further questions, contact a qualified exercise professional.

PARTICIPANT DECLARATION
If you are less than the legal age required for consent or require the assent of a care provider, your parent, guardian or care provider must also sign this form.

I, the undersigned, have read, understood to my full satisfaction and completed this questionnaire. I acknowledge that this physical activity clearance is valid for a maximum of 12 months from the date it is completed and becomes invalid if my condition changes. I also acknowledge that the community/fitness center may retain a copy of this form for its records. In these instances, it will maintain the confidentiality of the same, complying with applicable law.

NAME _____ DATE _____

SIGNATURE _____ WITNESS_____

SIGNATURE OF PARENT/GUARDIAN/CARE PROVIDER _____

⬤ **If you answered YES to one or more of the questions above, COMPLETE PAGES 2 AND 3.**

⚠ **Delay becoming more active if:**
- ✓ You have a temporary illness such as a cold or fever; it is best to wait until you feel better.
- ✓ You are pregnant - talk to your health care practitioner, your physician, a qualified exercise professional, and/or complete the ePARmed-X+ at www.eparmedx.com before becoming more physically active.
- ✓ Your health changes - answer the questions on Pages 2 and 3 of this document and/or talk to your doctor or a qualified exercise professional before continuing with any physical activity program.

2023 PAR-Q+

FOLLOW-UP QUESTIONS ABOUT YOUR MEDICAL CONDITION(S)

1.	**Do you have Arthritis, Osteoporosis, or Back Problems?**	
	If the above condition(s) is/are present, answer questions 1a-1c If **NO** ☐ go to question 2	
1a.	Do you have difficulty controlling your condition with medications or other physician-prescribed therapies? (Answer **NO** if you are not currently taking medications or other treatments)	YES ☐ NO ☐
1b.	Do you have joint problems causing pain, a recent fracture or fracture caused by osteoporosis or cancer, displaced vertebra (e.g., spondylolisthesis), and/or spondylolysis/pars defect (a crack in the bony ring on the back of the spinal column)?	YES ☐ NO ☐
1c.	Have you had steroid injections or taken steroid tablets regularly for more than 3 months?	YES ☐ NO ☐
2.	**Do you currently have Cancer of any kind?**	
	If the above condition(s) is/are present, answer questions 2a-2b If **NO** ☐ go to question 3	
2a.	Does your cancer diagnosis include any of the following types: lung/bronchogenic, multiple myeloma (cancer of plasma cells), head, and/or neck?	YES ☐ NO ☐
2b.	Are you currently receiving cancer therapy (such as chemotheraphy or radiotherapy)?	YES ☐ NO ☐
3.	**Do you have a Heart or Cardiovascular Condition? This includes Coronary Artery Disease, Heart Failure, Diagnosed Abnormality of Heart Rhythm**	
	If the above condition(s) is/are present, answer questions 3a-3d If **NO** ☐ go to question 4	
3a.	Do you have difficulty controlling your condition with medications or other physician-prescribed therapies? (Answer **NO** if you are not currently taking medications or other treatments)	YES ☐ NO ☐
3b.	Do you have an irregular heart beat that requires medical management? (e.g., atrial fibrillation, premature ventricular contraction)	YES ☐ NO ☐
3c.	Do you have chronic heart failure?	YES ☐ NO ☐
3d.	Do you have diagnosed coronary artery (cardiovascular) disease and have not participated in regular physical activity in the last 2 months?	YES ☐ NO ☐
4.	**Do you currently have High Blood Pressure?**	
	If the above condition(s) is/are present, answer questions 4a-4b If **NO** ☐ go to question 5	
4a.	Do you have difficulty controlling your condition with medications or other physician-prescribed therapies? (Answer **NO** if you are not currently taking medications or other treatments)	YES ☐ NO ☐
4b.	Do you have a resting blood pressure equal to or greater than 160/90 mmHg with or without medication? (Answer **YES** if you do not know your resting blood pressure)	YES ☐ NO ☐
5.	**Do you have any Metabolic Conditions? This includes Type 1 Diabetes, Type 2 Diabetes, Pre-Diabetes**	
	If the above condition(s) is/are present, answer questions 5a-5e If **NO** ☐ go to question 6	
5a.	Do you often have difficulty controlling your blood sugar levels with foods, medications, or other physician- prescribed therapies?	YES ☐ NO ☐
5b.	Do you often suffer from signs and symptoms of low blood sugar (hypoglycemia) following exercise and/or during activities of daily living? Signs of hypoglycemia may include shakiness, nervousness, unusual irritability, abnormal sweating, dizziness or light-headedness, mental confusion, difficulty speaking, weakness, or sleepiness.	YES ☐ NO ☐
5c.	Do you have any signs or symptoms of diabetes complications such as heart or vascular disease and/or complications affecting your eyes, kidneys, **OR** the sensation in your toes and feet?	YES ☐ NO ☐
5d.	Do you have other metabolic conditions (such as current pregnancy-related diabetes, chronic kidney disease, or liver problems)?	YES ☐ NO ☐
5e.	Are you planning to engage in what for you is unusually high (or vigorous) intensity exercise in the near future?	YES ☐ NO ☐

2023 PAR-Q+

6. Do you have any Mental Health Problems or Learning Difficulties? This includes Alzheimer's, Dementia, Depression, Anxiety Disorder, Eating Disorder, Psychotic Disorder, Intellectual Disability, Down Syndrome

If the above condition(s) is/are present, answer questions 6a-6b   If **NO** ☐ go to question 7

6a.	Do you have difficulty controlling your condition with medications or other physician-prescribed therapies? (Answer **NO** if you are not currently taking medications or other treatments)	YES ☐	NO ☐
6b.	Do you have Down Syndrome AND back problems affecting nerves or muscles?	YES ☐	NO ☐

7. Do you have a Respiratory Disease? This includes Chronic Obstructive Pulmonary Disease, Asthma, Pulmonary High Blood Pressure

If the above condition(s) is/are present, answer questions 7a-7d   If **NO** ☐ go to question 8

7a.	Do you have difficulty controlling your condition with medications or other physician-prescribed therapies? (Answer **NO** if you are not currently taking medications or other treatments)	YES ☐	NO ☐
7b.	Has your doctor ever said your blood oxygen level is low at rest or during exercise and/or that you require supplemental oxygen therapy?	YES ☐	NO ☐
7c.	If asthmatic, do you currently have symptoms of chest tightness, wheezing, laboured breathing, consistent cough (more than 2 days/week), or have you used your rescue medication more than twice in the last week?	YES ☐	NO ☐
7d.	Has your doctor ever said you have high blood pressure in the blood vessels of your lungs?	YES ☐	NO ☐

8. Do you have a Spinal Cord Injury? This includes Tetraplegia and Paraplegia

If the above condition(s) is/are present, answer questions 8a-8c   If **NO** ☐ go to question 9

8a.	Do you have difficulty controlling your condition with medications or other physician-prescribed therapies? (Answer **NO** if you are not currently taking medications or other treatments)	YES ☐	NO ☐
8b.	Do you commonly exhibit low resting blood pressure significant enough to cause dizziness, light-headedness, and/or fainting?	YES ☐	NO ☐
8c.	Has your physician indicated that you exhibit sudden bouts of high blood pressure (known as Autonomic Dysreflexia)?	YES ☐	NO ☐

9. Have you had a Stroke? This includes Transient Ischemic Attack (TIA) or Cerebrovascular Event

If the above condition(s) is/are present, answer questions 9a-9c   If **NO** ☐ go to question 10

9a.	Do you have difficulty controlling your condition with medications or other physician-prescribed therapies? (Answer NO if you are not currently taking medications or other treatments)	YES ☐	NO ☐
9b.	Do you have any impairment in walking or mobility?	YES ☐	NO ☐
9c.	Have you experienced a stroke or impairment in nerves or muscles in the past 6 months?	YES ☐	NO ☐

10. Do you have any other medical condition not listed above or do you have two or more medical conditions?

If you have other medical conditions, answer questions 10a-10c   If **NO** ☐ read the Page 4 recommendations

10a.	Have you experienced a blackout, fainted, or lost consciousness as a result of a head injury within the last 12 months OR have you had a diagnosed concussion within the last 12 months?	YES ☐	NO ☐
10b.	Do you have a medical condition that is not listed (such as epilepsy, neurological conditions, kidney problems)?	YES ☐	NO ☐
10c.	Do you currently live with two or more medical conditions?	YES ☐	NO ☐

PLEASE LIST YOUR MEDICAL CONDITION(S) AND ANY RELATED MEDICATIONS HERE: _____

_____

_____

GO to Page 4 for recommendations about your current medical condition(s) and sign the PARTICIPANT DECLARATION.

2023 PAR-Q+

☑ **If you answered NO to all of the FOLLOW-UP questions (pgs. 2-3) about your medical condition, you are ready to become more physically active - sign the PARTICIPANT DECLARATION below:**
- ▶ It is advised that you consult a qualified exercise professional to help you develop a safe and effective physical activity plan to meet your health needs.
- ▶ You are encouraged to start slowly and build up gradually - 20 to 60 minutes of low to moderate intensity exercise, 3-5 days per week including aerobic and muscle strengthening exercises.
- ▶ As you progress, you should aim to accumulate 150 minutes or more of moderate intensity physical activity per week.
- ▶ If you are over the age of 45 yr and **NOT** accustomed to regular vigorous to maximal effort exercise, consult a qualified exercise professional before engaging in this intensity of exercise.

⬤ If you answered **YES** to **one or more of the follow-up questions** about your medical condition: You should seek further information before becoming more physically active or engaging in a fitness appraisal. You should complete the specially designed online screening and exercise recommendations program - the **ePARmed-X+ at www.eparmedx.com** and/or visit a qualified exercise professional to work through the ePARmed-X+ and for further information.

⚠ **Delay becoming more active if:**
- ✓ You have a temporary illness such as a cold or fever; it is best to wait until you feel better.
- ✓ You are pregnant - talk to your health care practitioner, your physician, a qualified exercise professional, and/or complete the ePARmed-X+ **at www.eparmedx.com** before becoming more physically active.
- ✓ Your health changes - talk to your doctor or qualified exercise professional before continuing with any physical activity program.

- You are encouraged to photocopy the PAR-Q+. You must use the entire questionnaire and NO changes are permitted.
- The authors, the PAR-Q+ Collaboration, partner organizations, and their agents assume no liability for persons who undertake physical activity and/or make use of the PAR-Q+ or ePARmed-X+. If in doubt after completing the questionnaire, consult your doctor prior to physical activity.

PARTICIPANT DECLARATION

- All persons who have completed the PAR-Q+ please read and sign the declaration below.
- If you are less than the legal age required for consent or require the assent of a care provider, your parent, guardian or care provider must also sign this form.

I, the undersigned, have read, understood to my full satisfaction and completed this questionnaire. I acknowledge that this physical activity clearance is valid for a maximum of 12 months from the date it is completed and becomes invalid if my condition changes. I also acknowledge that the community/fitness center may retain a copy of this form for its records. In these instances, it will maintain the confidentiality of the same, complying with applicable law.

NAME _____ DATE _____

SIGNATURE _____ WITNESS_____

SIGNATURE OF PARENT/GUARDIAN/CARE PROVIDER _____

――――――――――― For more information, please contact ―――――――――――

www.eparmedx.com

Email: eparmedx@gmail.com

Citation for PAR-Q+
Warburton DER, Jamnik VK, Bredin SSD, and Gledhill N on behalf of the PAR-Q+ Collaboration. The Physical Activity Readiness Questionnaire for Everyone (PAR-Q+) and Electronic Physical Activity Readiness Medical Examination (ePARmed-X+). Health & Fitness Journal of Canada 4(2):3-23, 2011.

The PAR-Q+ was created using the evidence-based AGREE process (1) by the PAR-Q+ Collaboration chaired by Dr. Darren E. R. Warburton with Dr. Norman Gledhill, Dr. Veronica Jamnik, and Dr. Donald C. McKenzie (2). Production of this document has been made possible through financial contributions from the Public Health Agency of Canada and the BC Ministry of Health Services. The views expressed herein do not necessarily represent the views of the Public Health Agency of Canada or the BC Ministry of Health Services.

Key References
1. Jamnik VK, Warburton DER, Makarski J, McKenzie DC, Shephard RJ, Stone J, and Gledhill N. Enhancing the effectiveness of clearance for physical activity participation; background and overall process. APNM 36(S1):S3-S13, 2011.
2. Warburton DER, Gledhill N, Jamnik VK, Bredin SSD, McKenzie DC, Stone J, Charlesworth S, and Shephard RJ. Evidence-based risk assessment and recommendations for physical activity clearance; Consensus Document. APNM 36(S1):S266-s298, 2011.
3. Chisholm DM, Collis ML, Kulak LL, Davenport W, and Gruber N. Physical activity readiness. British Columbia Medical Journal. 1975;17:375-378.
4. Thomas S, Reading J, and Shephard RJ. Revision of the Physical Activity Readiness Questionnaire (PAR-Q). Canadian Journal of Sport Science 1992;17:4 338-345.

CONCLUSION

In conclusion, there is a pressing need to promote, recommend, and prescribe exercise therapy in prostate cancer care. It has been proven to be tolerable, safe, and linked to improved physical, mental, and social wellbeing. Physiotherapists must carefully design and individualize exercise parameters during exercise therapy sessions. In general, exercise programs must include cardiovascular, resistance, balance, flexibility, and functional training. Vigorous activities must be implemented for at least 75 minutes a week, and strength training of all major muscle groups (with special consideration given to bone metastatic cancer patients) must be performed at least twice a week. Power training (performing concentric action as quickly as possible and eccentric action within 2–3 seconds) may also benefit the older population in improving physical function. A comprehensive pre-surgical exercise program should be administered to those waiting to have prostatectomy surgery to prevent muscle loss post-surgery and to improve surgical outcomes.

For those with cardiovascular risks, screening and risk assessments may need to be performed during cancer treatments to determine the safest and most effective exercise therapy prescription. Specialized prostate cancer group exercise programs may help improve adherence, create a positive environment, and increase the perception of wellness.

Exercise therapy is likely the best form of medicine that acts on multiple systems to improve quality of life, restore function, prevent frailty, and reduce side-effects of prostate cancer treatments.

EXERCISE RESOURCES FOR PROSTATE CANCER SURVIVORS
Australia
PROST!: www.prost.com.au

Canada
Prostate Cancer Supportive Care Program, Vancouver, CA: https://pcscprogram.ca

Alberta Cancer Exercise: www.albertacancerexercise.com

SIRvivor BC: Prostate Cancer Exercise Program: https://www.bcrpa.bc.ca/everything-else/sirvivor-bc/

TrueNTH: https://lifestyle.truenth.ca

UW WELL-FIT cancer exercise programs: https://uwaterloo.ca/health/uw-well-fit

USA

Fred Hutchinson Cancer Center: www.fredhutch.org/en/research/institutes-networks-ircs/institute-for-prostate-cancer-research/patient-video-series.html

Cancer.Net—Exercise routine for men with prostate cancer: www.cancer.net/survivorship/healthy-living/exercise-during-cancer-treatment

REFERENCES

2018 Physical Activity Guidelines Advisory Committee (2018). *Physical Activity Guidelines Advisory Committee Scientific Report*. Washington D.C.: US Department of Health and Human Services, 779.

Ainsworth, B.E., Haskell, W.L., Whitt, M.C., Irwin, M.L., *et al.* (n.d.). *Compendium of Physical Activities*. Retrieved July 4, 2022, from https://sites.google.com/site/compendiumofphysicalactivities

Alder, R., Zetner, D., & Rosenberg, J. (2020). Incidence of inguinal hernia after radical prostatectomy: A systematic review and meta-analysis. *Journal of Urology, 203*(2), 265–274. https://doi.org/10.1097/JU.0000000000000313

Ashton, R.E., Aning, J.J., Tew, G.A., Robson, W.A., & Saxton, J.M. (2021). Supported progressive resistance exercise training to counter the adverse side-effects of robot-assisted radical prostatectomy: A randomised controlled trial. *Supportive Care in Cancer, 29*(8), 4595–4605. https://doi.org/10.1007/s00520-021-06002-5

Balachandran, A.T., Steele, J., Angielczyk, D., Belio, M., *et al.* (2022). Comparison of power training vs traditional strength training on physical function in older adults: A systematic review and meta-analysis. *JAMA Network Open, 5*(5), e2211623. https://doi.org/10.1001/jamanetworkopen.2022.11623

Barranquero, A.G., Tobaruela, E., Bajawi, M., Muñoz, P., Die Trill, J., & Garcia-Perez, J.C. (2020). Incidence and risk factors for incisional hernia after temporary loop ileostomy closure: Choosing candidates for prophylactic mesh placement. *Hernia, 24*(1), 93–98. https://doi.org/10.1007/s10029-019-02042-3

Baumann, F.T., Zopf, E.M., Bloch, W., Baumann, F.T., Zopf, E.M., & Bloch, W. (2012). Clinical exercise interventions in prostate cancer patients—A systematic review of randomized controlled trials. *Supportive Care in Cancer, 20*(2), 221–233. https://doi.org/10.1007/s00520-011-1271-0

Betof, A.S., Dewhirst, M.W., & Jones, L.W. (2013). Effects and potential mechanisms of exercise training on cancer progression: A translational perspective. *Brain, Behavior, and Immunity, 30 Suppl*, S75-87. https://doi.org/10.1016/j.bbi.2012.05.001

Betof, A.S., Lascola, C.D., Weitzel, D., Landon, C., *et al.* (2015). Modulation of murine breast tumor vascularity, hypoxia and chemotherapeutic response by exercise. *Journal of the National Cancer Institute, 107*(5), djv040. https://doi.org/10.1093/jnci/djv040

Bhatia, N., Santos, M., Jones, L.W., Beckman, J.A., Penson, D.F., Morgans, A.K., & Moslehi, J. (2016). Cardiovascular effects of androgen deprivation therapy for the treatment of prostate cancer: ABCDE steps to reduce cardiovascular disease in patients with prostate cancer. *Circulation, 133*(5), 537–541. https://doi.org/10.1161/CIRCULATIONAHA.115.012519

Bonsignore, A., Marwick, T.H., Adams, S.C., Thampinathan, B., *et al.* (2021). Clinical, echocardiographic, and biomarker associations with impaired cardiorespiratory fitness early after HER2-targeted breast cancer therapy. *JACC: CardioOncology, 3*(5), 678–691. https://doi.org/10.1016/j.jaccao.2021.08.010

Borde, R., Hortobágyi, T., & Granacher, U. (2015). Dose-response relationships of resistance training in healthy old adults: A systematic review and meta-analysis. *Sports Medicine (Auckland, N.Z.), 45*(12), 1693–1720. https://doi.org/10.1007/s40279-015-0385-9

Campbell, C.M., Zhang, K.W., Collier, A., Linch, M., *et al.* (2020). Cardiovascular complications of prostate cancer therapy. *Current Treatment Options in Cardiovascular Medicine, 22*(12), 1–27. https://doi.org/10.1007/s11936-020-00873-3

Carrasco, C., Tomas-Carus, P., Bravo, J., Pereira, C., & Mendes, F. (2020). Understanding fall risk factors in community-dwelling older adults: A cross-sectional study. *International Journal of Older People Nursing, 15*(1), e12294. https://doi.org/10.1111/opn.12294

Chung, K.H., Park, S.B., Streckmann, F., Wiskemann, J., *et al.* (2022). Mechanisms, mediators, and moderators of the effects of exercise on chemotherapy-induced peripheral neuropathy. *Cancers, 14*(5), Article 5. https://doi.org/10.3390/cancers14051224

Cormie, P., Newton, R.U., Spry, N., Joseph, D., Taaffe, D.R., & Galvão, D.A. (2013). Safety and efficacy of resistance exercise in prostate cancer patients with bone metastases. *Prostate Cancer and Prostatic Diseases, 16*(4), 328–335. https://doi.org/10.1038/pcan.2013.22

Cormie, P., Turner, B., Kaczmarek, E., Drake, D., & Chambers, S.K. (2015). A qualitative exploration of the experience of men with prostate cancer involved in supervised exercise programs. *Oncology Nursing Forum, 42*(1), 24–32. https://doi.org/10.1188/15.ONF.24-32

Danhauer, S.C., Addington, E.L., Sohl, S.J., Chaoul, A., & Cohen, L. (2017). Review of yoga therapy during cancer treatment. *Supportive Care in Cancer, 25*(4), 1357–1372. https://doi.org/10.1007/s00520-016-3556-9

Fox, L., Wiseman, T., Cahill, D., Beyer, K., Peat, N., Rammant, E., & Van Hemelrijck, M. (2019). Barriers and facilitators to physical activity in men with prostate cancer: A qualitative and quantitative systematic review. *Psycho-Oncology, 28*(12), 2270–2285. https://doi.org/10.1002/pon.5240

Harrington, J.M., Schwenke, D.C., & Epstein, D.R. (2013). Exercise preferences among men with prostate cancer receiving androgen-deprivation therapy. *Oncology Nursing Forum, 40*(5), E358–367. https://doi.org/10.1188/13.ONF.E358-E367

Jones, L.W., Eves, N.D., & Peppercorn, J. (2010). Pre-exercise screening and prescription guidelines for cancer patients. *The Lancet Oncology, 11*(10), 914–916. https://doi.org/10.1016/S1470-2045(10)70184-4

Jordan, B.F., & Sonveaux, P. (2012). Targeting tumor perfusion and oxygenation to improve the outcome of anticancer therapy. *Frontiers in Pharmacology, 3*, 94. https://doi.org/10.3389/fphar.2012.00094

Kang, D.-W., Fairey, A.S., Boulé, N.G., Field, C.J., Wharton, S.A., & Courneya, K.S. (2021). Effects of exercise on cardiorespiratory fitness and biochemical progression in men with localized prostate cancer under active surveillance: The ERASE randomized clinical trial. *JAMA Oncology, 7*(10), 1487–1495. https://doi.org/10.1001/jamaoncol.2021.3067

Kang, D.-W., Fairey, A.S., Boulé, N.G., Field, C.J., Wharton, S.A., & Courneya, K.S. (2022). A randomized trial of the effects of exercise on anxiety, fear of cancer progression and quality of life in prostate cancer patients on active surveillance. *Journal of Urology, 207*(4), 814–822. https://doi.org/10.1097/JU.0000000000002334

Kokkonen, J., Nelson, A.G., Eldredge, C., & Winchester, J.B. (2007). Chronic static stretching improves exercise performance. *Medicine & Science in Sports & Exercise, 39*(10), 1825–1831. https://doi.org/10.1249/mss.0b013e3181238a2b

Mahfouz, M., & Al-Juaid, R. (2021). Prevalence and risk factors of abdominal hernia among Saudi population. *Journal of Family Medicine & Primary Care, 10*(8), 3130–3136. https://doi.org/10.4103/jfmpc.jfmpc_622_21

Moustafa, I.M., Ahbouch, A., Palakkottuparambil, F., & Walton, L.M. (2021). Optimal duration of stretching of the hamstring muscle group in older adults: A randomized controlled trial. *European Journal of Physical and Rehabilitation Medicine, 57*(6), 931–939. https://doi.org/10.23736/S1973-9087.21.06731-9

Paltiel, H., Solvoll, E., Loge, J.H., Kaasa, S., & Oldervoll, L. (2009). "The healthy me appears": Palliative cancer patients' experiences of participation in a physical group exercise program. *Palliative & Supportive Care, 7*(4), 459–467. https://doi.org/10.1017/S1478951509990460

Pernar, C.H., Ebot, E.M., Pettersson, A., Graff, R.E., et al. (2019). A prospective study of the association between physical activity and risk of prostate cancer defined by clinical features and TMPRSS2:ERG. *European Urology, 76*(1), 33-40. https://doi.org/10.1016/j.eururo.2018.09.041

Pollock, M.L., Gaesser, G.A., Butcher, J.D., Després, J.-P., et al. (1998). ACSM position stand: The recommended quantity and quality of exercise for developing and maintaining cardiorespiratory and muscular fitness, and flexibility in healthy adults. *Medicine & Science in Sports & Exercise, 30*(6), 975-991.

Rock, C.L., Doyle, C., Demark-Wahnefried, W., Meyerhardt, J., et al. (2012). Nutrition and physical activity guidelines for cancer survivors. *CA: A Cancer Journal for Clinicians, 62*(4), 243-274. https://doi.org/10.3322/caac.21142

Schadler, K.L., Thomas, N.J., Galie, P.A., Bhang, D.H., et al. (2016). Tumor vessel normalization after aerobic exercise enhances chemotherapeutic efficacy. *Oncotarget, 7*(40), 65429-65440. https://doi.org/10.18632/oncotarget.11748

Schumacher, O., Galvão, D.A., Taaffe, D.R., Spry, N., et al. (2021). Effect of exercise adjunct to radiation and androgen deprivation therapy on patient-reported treatment toxicity in men with prostate cancer: A secondary analysis of 2 randomized controlled trials. *Practical Radiation Oncology, 11*(3), 215-225. https://doi.org/10.1016/j.prro.2021.01.005

Seguin, R., & Nelson, M.E. (2003). The benefits of strength training for older adults. *American Journal of Preventive Medicine, 25*(3 Suppl 2), 141-149. https://doi.org/10.1016/s0749-3797(03)00177-6

Singh, F., Newton, R.U., Baker, M.K., Spry, N.A., Taaffe, D.R., Thavaseelan, J., & Galvão, D.A. (2017). Feasibility of presurgical exercise in men with prostate cancer undergoing prostatectomy. *Integrative Cancer Therapies, 16*(3), 290-299. https://doi.org/10.1177/1534735416666373

Wall, B.A., Galvão, D.A., Fatehee, N., Taaffe, D.R., et al. (2017). Exercise improves V˙O2max and body composition in androgen deprivation therapy-treated prostate cancer patients. *Medicine & Science in Sports & Exercise, 49*(8), 1503-1510. https://doi.org/10.1249/MSS.0000000000001277

Waryasz, G.R. (2010). Exercise strategies to prevent the development of the anterior pelvic tilt: Implications for possible prevention of sports hernias and osteitis pubis. *Strength & Conditioning Journal, 32*(4), 56-65. https://doi.org/10.1519/SSC.0b013e3181d58aac

Wollesen, B., Mattes, K., Schulz, S., Bischoff, L.L., Seydell, L., Bell, J.W., & von Duvillard, S.P. (2017). Effects of Dual-Task Management and Resistance Training on Gait Performance in Older Individuals: A Randomized Controlled Trial. *Frontiers in Aging Neuroscience, 9*, 1-12. https://doi.org/10.3389/fnagi.2017.00415

Yang, L., Morielli, A.R., Heer, E., Kirkham, A.A., et al. (2021). Effects of exercise on cancer treatment efficacy: A systematic review of preclinical and clinical studies. *Cancer Research, 81*(19), 4889-4895. https://doi.org/10.1158/0008-5472.CAN-21-1258

Zoth, N., Tomanek, A., Seuthe, K., Pfister, R., & Baumann, F.T. (2023). Exercise as medicine could be a chance for early detection and prevention of Cardiotoxicity in cancer treatments - a narrative review. *Oncology Research and Treatment, 46*(4), 131-139. https://doi.org/10.1159/000529205

CHAPTER 9

Psychological Health

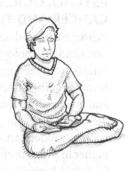

Psychological health—also known as mental health, emotional wellness, psychological resilience, mental stability, mental wellbeing, or emotional balance—is essential for the survivorship of prostate cancer patients. Psychological health's value has been so undermined and linked to so many taboos that even nowadays it can be a topic of reservation, discrimination, and dismissal from patients receiving care and their healthcare providers. Fortunately, its appreciation in the medical community has been increasing, as growing evidence suggests a correlation between psychological health status, physical health, and disease.[1] Although the understanding of the synergy between mental and physical health is improving, poor screening frequency, lack of referrals to psychology practices, and underestimation of mental health issues are still common subjects of concern in physiotherapy practices.[2] It is no small wonder that one of the key goals highlighted by the National Cancer Survivorship Initiative (NCSI) was to better address the psychological distress caused by the diagnosis and treatment of cancer.[3]

As described by the World Health Organization (WHO), psychological health (mental health) "is a state of mental wellbeing that enables people to cope with the stresses of life, realise their abilities, learn well and work well, and contribute to their community." Furthermore, the WHO describes mental health as much more than the absence of a mental illness, but a basic human right that is essential for individuals' decision making, relationship building, and shaping the world they live in.[4]

As psychological health is such a vast theme, this chapter's goal is to increase its awareness by introducing pertinent psychological health topics associated with prostate cancer survivors and their healthcare professionals. More specifically, it will raise appreciation for better understanding and

---

1   (Levine *et al.*, 2021)
2   (Heywood *et al.*, 2022)
3   (Watts *et al.*, 2014)
4   (World Health Organization, n.d.)

addressing psychological concerns related to the diagnosis and treatment of prostate cancer. It will introduce: the physiology of stress and its association with cancer; research findings on risks; the relationship of mental health disorders with prostate cancer and treatments symptoms and side-effects; healthcare clinicians' management and prevention of burnout and compassion fatigue; psychological health screening tools; and approaches and intervention suggestions.

PSYCHOLOGICAL HEALTH IN PROSTATE CANCER AND TREATMENTS

Prostate cancer diagnosis and treatment can trigger a wide variety of emotions and psychological responses in patients, friends, and family members. Emotions or feelings such as overwhelm, fear, grief, anger, frustration, helplessness, guilt, sadness, and worry are normal behavior after cancer diagnosis, and are usually transient in nature.[5] Occasionally, these feelings can become persistent, resulting in permanent mood changes or psychological distress such as anxiety and depression. Anxiety and depression are shown to be higher in prostate cancer survivors compared to non-cancer male population (2–3-fold higher), ranging from 15 percent to 27 percent peaking prior to and after the completion of treatment.[6] Clinically significant depression was reported in 8.2 percent to 36 percent of prostate cancer survivors, and its risks increase with previous diagnosis of anxiety and depression, younger age, smoking, former alcohol use, inability to perform work activities, and high risk prostate cancer.[7] Furthermore, coexisting depression and anxiety impact prostate cancer survivors' functional outcome and mortality.[8]

In addition to anxiety and depression, stress is commonly experienced during prostate cancer diagnosis and treatment, and can affect survivors' lives as well as cancer progression. Stress activates the sympathetic nervous system and the release of glucocorticoids, catecholamines, and other neuroendocrine factors, which have been associated with affecting immune processes relevant to tumor surveillance and containment, and encouraging cancer progression and metastasis.[9] Stress, depression, and anxiety have also been linked to downregulation of cellular immune responses, via depression of natural killer (NK) and T cell activities, which are normally defensors of cancer cells.[10] It has been hypothesized too that inflammation caused by tumor growth or treatment such as chemotherapy can affect the central nervous system,

---

5   (National Cancer Institute, 2014)
6   (Watts et al., 2014)
7   (Fervaha et al., 2020)
8   (Dinesh et al., 2021)
9   (Costanzo et al., 2011)
10 (Costanzo et al., 2011)

promoting depressive mood, fatigue, anorexia, pain, sleep disturbance, impaired concentration, and reduced activity.[11]

The diagnosis of prostate cancer and the side-effects of its treatments can present challenges to survivors' sense of masculinity, self-esteem, and body image. According to Bowie and colleagues' study, loss of sexual function, and libido after androgen deprivation therapy (ADT) and prostatectomy surgery were the most important life changes affecting men's sense of "manhood", body image, and self-esteem. This study also demonstrated that fatigue, urinary incontinence, removal of the prostate, and a loss of ownership over their bodies had an effect on body image, resulting in men perceiving their body as deficient and less than whole. Loss of ownership caused by increased healthcare consultations, tests, and body "handling" also increased a sense of vulnerability and shame.[12]

The diagnosis of prostate cancer and its treatment effects can challenge men's ideals of masculinity, particularly for those who subscribe to traditional hegemonic masculine norms. These norms include beliefs in heterosexism, power, self-sufficiency, restricted emotional expression, misogyny, and stoicism.[13] Hegemonic masculine ideals may have implications for men's mental wellbeing and adjustment post-prostate cancer diagnosis. Men who show inflexibility on their views of masculinity and sexual role may be more distressed when presented with changes post-treatment, compared to the ones with more flexible ideals.[14]

On a positive note, optimism was shown to improve health-related quality of life (HrQL) before prostate cancer biopsy results, and self-efficacy to improve HrQL after prostate cancer diagnosis and treatment was chosen.[15]

PSYCHOLOGICAL HEALTH AND THE BLADDER

The bladder can be a very "emotional" organ, reacting to stress, anxiety, and depression. Many studies have linked a relationship between urinary incontinence, urgency, and bladder pain to depression and anxiety.[16, 17, 18, 19, 20] A large population-based survey study was able to show that depression and anxiety are risk factors for developing urinary incontinence and that urinary incontinence may be associated with increased risk of depression and

11   (Costanzo et al., 2011)
12   (Bowie et al., 2022)
13   (Wall & Kristjanson, 2005)
14   (Bowie et al., 2022)
15   (Cuypers et al., 2018)
16   (Perry et al., 2006)
17   (Watkins et al., 2011)
18   (McKernan et al., 2018)
19   (Lai et al., 2016)
20   (Zorn et al., 1999)

anxiety.[21] Stress also appears to play a role in lower urinary tract symptoms such as painful bladder syndromes and overactive bladder.[22]

Prostate cancer survivors with increased urinary symptoms can increase the risk of developing anxiety and depression, and on the other hand, depression may increase their likelihood of urinary symptoms and decreased function outcomes.[23] Urinary incontinence can affect men's emotional and social wellbeing in great regards, contributing to increased feelings of anxiety, frustration, embarrassment, and depression, resulting in social isolation and decreased activity and participation.[24, 25]

Given that prostate cancer survivors are at risk for developing bladder symptoms, as well as depression and anxiety, and that urinary incontinence can highly affect men's emotional wellbeing, psychological screening and interventions should be highly regarded and part of their treatment plan.

PSYCHOLOGICAL HEALTH ASSESSMENT TOOLS
Questionnaires

Screening tools for psychological health can aid in identifying both mental distress among prostate cancer survivors and the impact of side-effects, such as urinary incontinence. However, screening questionnaires' sensitivities may not be as high in cancer patients. As an example, Osório and colleagues' study found about 50 percent false negative rates in cancer patients using the PHQ-4D (Patient Health Questionnaire) for depression and Generalized Anxiety Disorder Screener (GAD-7) for anxiety screening.[26] Esser and colleagues recommended different cut-offs when using the Hospital Anxiety and Depression Scale (HADS) and GAD-7 in cancer patients, due to lower sensitivities in officially recommended thresholds.[27] Lower sensitivities could be attributed to higher distress perceived by cancer patients during the adjustment to the disease that could be transient in nature, or comorbidity symptoms experienced by cancer survivors that may overlap with psychiatric symptoms.[28] Therefore, as well as administering questionnaires, fostering strong therapeutic alliances (while providing prostate survivors a safe and collaborative space during clinical interactions) may give the clinicians more insight into survivors' psychological wellness, while encouraging survivors to express their emotions more accurately and promptly.

Here are a few examples of questionnaires that can be used to screen for depression, anxiety, and stress:

---

21 (Felde *et al.*, 2017)
22 (Smith *et al.*, 2011)
23 (Dinesh *et al.*, 2021)
24 (Teunissen *et al.*, 2006)
25 (Bedretdinova *et al.*, 2016)
26 (Osório *et al.*, 2015)
27 (Esser *et al.*, 2018)
28 (Osório *et al.*, 2015)

- *International Consultation on Incontinence Questionnaire short-form (ICIQ-SF)*: The ICIQ-SF (see Figure 9.1) can be used by clinicians and researchers to assess the severity of urinary incontinence and its impact on quality of life.[29] The ICIQ-SF was shown to be valid, reliable, and responsive to change when assessing changes in urinary leakage and interference with everyday life activities.[30] The total score ranges from a low of 0 to a high of 21; the higher the score, the greater the level of incontinence and higher the burden on quality of life.
- *HADS*: The Hospital Anxiety and Depression Scale has been widely used in prostate cancer research. It has been shown to be a valid and reliable tool for detecting anxiety and depression, cut-off suggestions being ≥ 8.[31]
- *PHQ-9*: This is a brief depression severity measure. It was shown to be valid and reliable, and could be a useful tool in clinical settings due to its brevity.[32] Cut-off recommended is ≥ 7.[33]
- *Center for Epidemiologic Studies Depression Scale (CESD)*: The CESD has been the most frequent scale used in prostate cancer research to assess depression.[34] It was created in 1977, and revised in 2004. The CESD has 20 items, measuring symptoms of depression in nine different groups: sadness, loss of interest, appetite, sleep, concentration, guilt (worthlessness), fatigue, agitation, and suicidal ideation.[35] It has been shown to be a valid and reliable tool, with a cut-off point of 16 or higher.[36] It is a tool that can be used for free as it is in the public domain.[37]
- *NCCN Distress Thermometer and Problem List (DTPL)*: The DTPL is available as a free resource in 71 different languages. It has been developed to "identify and address the unpleasant experiences that may make it harder to cope with having cancer, its symptoms, or treatment."[38] It can be a helpful tool to screen for emotional distress and suicide in cancer patients, a score of 3 having the highest sensitivity to rule out suicide ideation, and a score of 9 the highest specificity for suicide ideation.[39] For prostate cancer patients a cut-off of ≥ 4 may be optimal soon after diagnosis, and ≥ 3 for longer-term assessments.[40]

---

29 (ICIQ, n.d.)
30 (Avery *et al.*, 2004)
31 (Watts *et al.*, 2014)
32 (Kroenke *et al.*, 2001)
33 (Esser *et al.*, 2018)
34 (Chien *et al.*, 2014)
35 (The Center for Epidemiologic Studies Depression Scale (CESD), 2017)
36 (Saracino *et al.*, 2017)
37 https://cesd-r.com/about-cesdr
38 (National Comprehensive Cancer Network (NCCN), n.d.)
39 (Chiang *et al.*, 2022)
40 (Chambers *et al.*, 2014)

- *GAD-7*: This was shown to be an adequate diagnostic measure for screening anxiety in the cancer population; however, cut-offs may be lower (≥7).[41]

☐☐☐ ☐☐ ☐☐☐   ICIQ-UI Short Form   ☐☐ ☐☐ ☐☐

Initial number   **CONFIDENTIAL**   DAY MONTH YEAR

Today's date

Many people leak urine some of the time. We are trying to find out how many people leak urine, and how much this bothers them. We would be grateful if you could answer the following questions, thinking about how you have been, on average, over the PAST FOUR WEEKS.

1 Please write in your date of birth: ☐☐ ☐☐ ☐☐

DAY MONTH YEAR

2 Are you (tick one): Female Male   MALE ☐   FEMALE ☐

---

3 How often do you leak urine?

(Tick one box)

never	☐	0
about once a week or less often	☐	1
two or three times a week	☐	2
about once a day	☐	3
several times a day	☐	4
all the time	☐	5

---

4 We would like to know how much urine you think leaks. How much urine do you usually leak (whether you wear protection or not)?

(Tick one box)

none	☐	0
a small amount	☐	2
a moderate amount	☐	4
a large amount	☐	6

---

5 Overall, how much does leaking urine interfere with your everyday life?

0   1   2   3   4   5   6   7   8   9   10

not at all   a great deal

ICIQ score: sum scores 3+4+5 ☐☐

---

6 When does urine leak? (Please tick all that apply to you)

never – urine does not leak	☐
leaks before you can get to the toilet	☐
leaks when you cough or sneeze	☐
leaks when you are asleep	☐
leaks when you are physically active/exercising	☐
leaks when you have finished urinating and are dressed	☐
leaks for no obvious reason	☐
leaks all the time	☐

Thank you very much for answering these questions.

FIGURE 9.1: ICIQ-SF

Copyright © ICIQ Group

---

41 (Esser *et al.*, 2018)

NCCN Guidelines Version 2.2023
Distress Management

National
Comprehensive
Cancer
Network®

NCCN DISTRESS THERMOMETER

Distress is an unpleasant experience of a mental, physical, social, or spiritual nature. It can affect the way you think, feel, or act. Distress may make it harder to cope with having cancer, its symptoms, or its treatment.

Instructions: Please circle the number (0–10) that best describes how much distress you have been experiencing in the past week, including today.

Extreme distress
10
9
8
7
6
5
4
3
2
1
0
No distress

PROBLEM LIST

Have you had concerns about any of the items below in the past week, including today? (Mark all that apply)

PHYSICAL CONCERNS
☐ Pain
☐ Sleep
☐ Fatigue
☐ Tobacco use
☐ Substance use
☐ Memory or concentration
☐ Sexual health
☐ Changes in eating
☐ Loss or change of physical abilities

EMOTIONAL CONCERNS
☐ Worry or anxiety
☐ Sadness or depression
☐ Loss of interest or enjoyment
☐ Grief or loss
☐ Fear
☐ Loneliness
☐ Anger
☐ Changes in appearance
☐ Feelings of worthlessness or being a burden

SOCIAL CONCERNS
☐ Relationship with spouse or partner
☐ Relationship with children
☐ Relationship with family members
☐ Relationship with friends or coworkers
☐ Communication with health care team
☐ Ability to have children

PRACTICAL CONCERNS
☐ Taking care of myself
☐ Taking care of others
☐ Work
☐ School
☐ Housing
☐ Finances
☐ Insurance
☐ Transportation
☐ Child care
☐ Having enough food
☐ Access to medicine
☐ Treatment decisions

SPIRITUAL OR RELIGIOUS CONCERNS
☐ Sense of meaning or purpose
☐ Changes in faith or beliefs
☐ Death, dying, or afterlife
☐ Conflict between beliefs and cancer treatments
☐ Relationship with the sacred
☐ Ritual or dietary needs

OTHER CONCERNS

Note: All recommendations are category 2A unless otherwise indicated.
Clinical Trials: NCCN believes that the best management of any patient with cancer is in a clinical trial. Participation in clinical trials is especially encouraged.

FIGURE 9.2: NCCN DISTRESS THERMOMETER AND PROBLEM LIST

HOW TO PROCEED AFTER DISCLOSURE OF PSYCHOLOGICAL DISTRESS

Physiotherapists and healthcare professionals who are administering psychological health screening tools need to understand the clinical reasoning why they are being administered (within their scope of practice) and how to follow up, especially in emergency situations following distressing disclosures such as *suicidal ideation*. These processes should be in place in clinical or hospital settings, and professionals involved in direct cancer patient care should be aware of them. Processes can include familiarizing oneself with local mental health hospital services, crisis hotlines, community services, and professionals.

Many health professional colleges may be able to suggest strategies for clinicians to support clients during acute mental health crises. For example, colleges of physical therapists in Canada suggest being prepared to stop any physical treatment to support the client during a psychological crisis by offering kind words of acknowledgment, resources, and referrals to appropriate professionals.[42, 43] Crisis hotlines can be an excellent tool, and can be accessed together with the person in distress during the clinical consultation. In serious situations when risk of harm is high and there is a risk of serious bodily harm or death, the privacy law allows clinicians to alert family members, physicians, or police authorities, even without patients' consent.[44] Ideally, these courses of action should align with a strong therapeutic alliance and moral/ethical professional obligations in supporting patients' wellbeing and best interests.

Health professionals, including physiotherapists, may feel not well prepared to deal with distress disclosures. There are courses such as *psychological first aid* or *mental health first aid* that can teach strategies on how to become more resilient during stressful situations and to improve approaches when responding to mental health crises.

Heart rate variability (HRV)

Heart rate variability can be used as an indicator of health status, and linked to self-regulatory capacities, resilience, and psychological wellbeing.[45] Stress as a response to cancer diagnosis and life-altering events has been shown to alter the autonomic nervous system (ANS) by stimulating the sympathetic

---

42   (College of Physical Therapists of British Columbia (CPTBC), 2023)
43   (College of Physiotherapists of Ontario, n.d.)
44   (College of Physiotherapists of Alberta, n.d.)
45   (Spada *et al.*, 2022)

nervous system (SNS), altering cell and immune responses which can encourage cancer cell growth.[46] HRV is the fluctuation in time between heart beats, and can be used as a biomarker of optimal autonomic balance or best interplay from the parasympathetic and sympathetic nervous system.[47, 48] Excessive increased SNS can be picked up by non-invasive methods of HRV, and may be used to screen mental stress in prostate cancer patients.

Majerova and colleagues suggested that ECG should be evaluated for a minimum of five minutes and there should be a device that enables calculation of HRV from raw data, while eliminating presences of artefacts.[49]

Some devices used in recent HRV studies include emWave Pro Multi-user, First Beat, and Symbiofi.

PSYCHOLOGICAL HEALTH INTERVENTIONS AND STRATEGIES
Support, active listening, and therapeutic alliance

Physiotherapists and health professionals underestimate the emotional impact they have on their cancer patients. As previously discussed, health professionals play a critical role in prostate cancer survivors' psychological wellbeing. Although some clinicians or physicians may find they are not well equipped to address patients' psychological distresses, they may still be the first people whom cancer patients talk to about their cancer journey, frustrations, challenges, and emotional impact. Clinicians may help alleviate some of these emotions by providing compassionate care, empathy, and support. Based on studies conducted in the field of musculoskeletal physiotherapy, being responsive was the number one quality that describes being a "good" physiotherapist, according to their patients.[50] Being responsive involves actively listening to patients' needs and concerns, showing acceptance, and "being attentive, taking an interest in patients, communicating verbally and nonverbally, and validating patient experiences."[51]

Many studies were able to support the importance of building strong therapeutic alliances between health providers and patients in cancer care.[52] As an example, physicians' empathy can positively impact prostate cancer patients' anxiety, perceived sigma, and self-efficacy.[53] As well as positively influencing emotional outcomes, strong physician—patient working alliances can also improve treatment outcomes, patient satisfaction, and adherence

46 (Costanzo et al., 2011)
47 (Spada et al., 2022)
48 (Shaffer & Ginsberg, 2017)
49 (Majerova et al., 2022)
50 (Kleiner et al., 2021)
51 (Kleiner et al., 2021)
52 (Schnur & Montgomery, 2010)
53 (Yang et al., 2018)

to medical recommendations.[54] Responsiveness and active listening may help build strong therapeutic alliances and be an important component to alleviate psychological distress in prostate cancer survivorship.

Psychosocial therapy

Psychosocial therapy, such as cognitive behavioral interventions, informational and educational interventions, non-behavioral counseling or psychotherapy, and social support, can be used to treat prostate cancer survivors' psychological distresses, such as depression and anxiety.[55] Psychosocial interventions, particularly cognitive behavioral therapy (CBT), have been shown to be beneficial in improving prostate cancer-related fatigue.[56] Jacobsen and Jim's review outlined five types of psychosocial interventions which can reduce anxiety and depression in cancer care:[57]

Psychoeducation for new cancer patients

This comprises brief 15-minute therapy sessions with a counselor delivered to newly diagnosed cancer patients at time of initial consultation with the oncologist. This session includes giving recommendations to available support services and opportunity to discuss concerns and offer suggestions on how to cope.

Problem-solving therapy for distressed cancer patients against depression

These are ten weekly 90-minute therapy sessions focused on applying four key strategies: to better define their problems, to present a wide variety of solutions for their problems, to identify the best solution, and to follow up after implementation of this solution.

Stress management training for chemotherapy patients to prevent anxiety and depression

This program is based on instructing chemotherapy patients on three stress management coping mechanisms ("paced abdominal breathing, progressive muscle relaxation training with guided imagery, and use of coping self-statements"[58]) via print and audiovisual materials before and after the start of chemotherapy.

Cognitive therapy for depression in patients with metastatic cancer

This intervention consists of eight weekly 60- to 90-minute cognitive therapy sessions followed by three booster sessions at three-week intervals, focused

---

54 (Fuertes *et al.*, 2007)
55 (Chien *et al.*, 2014)
56 (McConkey, 2016)
57 (Jacobsen & Jim, 2008)
58 (Jacobsen & Jim, 2008)

on modifying dysfunctional or irrational thoughts about the cancer. This therapy goal is to foster realistic and positive attitudes towards patients' life and health circumstances.

Group cognitive behavioral therapy for cancer survivors
This group therapy consists of six weekly 90-minute sessions led by a psychiatrist and co-led by two cancer survivors. During the program, stress management techniques (progressive muscle relaxation and self-hypnosis), mental imagery, goal setting, planning, and achieving change are introduced.

"Slow things down": An interview with Paul Griggs MC, RCC, registered clinical counselor and clinical lead for the Prostate Cancer Supportive Care (PCSC) Program in British Columbia, Canada

What is the role of counseling during prostate cancer survivorship? What are the common concerns you see? When (before treatment, after treatment, at diagnosis) do you commonly see patients?

I usually see prostate cancer survivors (generally from the age of around 40 to over 80) shortly after their diagnosis, after their treatment, or after metastasis was identified. While the effects of prostate cancer is a typical topic to discuss, I often find that the issues we address are not about their specific medical condition and more about life issues around personal relationships, work and career, previous life trauma, and other emotional distresses that may have been exacerbated after a cancer diagnosis and treatment.

I have been advocating more for physicians and specialists in the province to start referring their patients as soon as diagnosis to support patients through the distress of a diagnosis and to support them through their decisions on treatment (which can be overwhelming). Counseling sessions and participating in our supportive care program can be used as a way to *slow things down*. Give men the chance to "digest" the news of being diagnosed with cancer, and make individualized decisions that make sense for them and their families. Most of the time, due to our fast-paced public medical system, men are given the diagnosis and expected to research treatment options on their own—which can be challenging. Counseling sessions are designed to support men and their families through some of the worry and anxiety that can often accompany a diagnosis.

Have you responded to many mental health crises or do you have systems or strategies in place? What are your recommendations to other health professionals (non-clinical counselors) following distressing disclosure or suicidal ideation?

I believe this is an important and sensitive topic in prostate cancer care. Responding to patient distress, which can include (although rarely) thoughts of self-harm, suicide, or "what is the point of living?" can be a very challenging experience, even for trained clinical counselors like myself. At the PCSC Program, we have a team of clinicians with different educational backgrounds (physiotherapists, sexual health nurses, and exercise specialists for example) who often are exposed to some of these potentially distressing disclosures. Hence, we are currently collaborating to implement systems and strategies to be better skilled if the circumstances arise.

Emotionally and operationally preparing staff members that are at risk of being faced with situations of distress may help to improve vulnerable patients' safety, improve therapeutic outcome and potentially reduce harm.

What are the main barriers in accessing counseling services (e.g., taboo from clients/health professionals, lack of understanding, lack of access, financial hardship)? What is your message to other health professionals who are treating this population—how can they integrate psychological-services awareness into their practices?

In my clinical experience I still see some social stigma attached to mental health services, especially if patients have never been to a counselor before. In my practice at the PCSC many patients come to me having never been to a counselor in the past. I can speculate that traditional *hegemonic masculine ideals* may influence men's attitude towards mental health counseling, impacting the likelihood in utilizing counseling as a resource for their emotional distress. The concept that men need to be "strong, resilient, and not express emotions" may be a barrier to being open to therapy. However, I do see men from all age groups who are open to or believe in the benefits of psychosocial therapy. I try to make their experiences positive during sessions, especially for those who are new to therapy. I try to understand their concepts of masculinity, asking questions such as "What are the main qualities that best define you as a man?", and at the same time challenging some of those concepts by reconstructing ideals of bravery or strength. I believe it requires strength for being vulnerable and open about your own emotional distress, or to explore different attitudes or coping mechanisms to improve psychological status.

Accessing counseling services in prostate cancer care may be challenging due to limited free access; for example, I am the only clinical counselor working at the PCSCP in the province, which can "potentially" serve approximately 100,000–140,000[59, 60] prostate cancer survivors. Our counseling services at the PCSC Program are free to BC (British Columbia)-resident prostate cancer patients; however, it can often have a waitlist and has a limited number of visits per patient. Counseling services in private care are readily available but it can be costly, especially for those who need ongoing support.

I find that *de-stigmatizing mental health* is what will increase the acceptance for psychosocial interventions, especially in cancer care.

Compared to other countries, what is your opinion on how Canada (BC) delivers services to prostate cancer survivors? What do you think we need, are lacking, or need improving, or what services need to be included for prostate cancer survivors in helping their mental health and quality of life?
I think we have innovative prostate cancer survivorship services here in BC. Although our public healthcare system faces challenges such as increased waitlists for specialized clinics and increased difficulty recruiting healthcare professionals for our growing aging population, I believe we are able to maintain quality services in prostate cancer care. As an example, the PCSC is a self-referred, research-based, free, comprehensive program for prostate cancer survivors, partners and families living in our province, from the time of initial diagnosis onwards. We offer educational and clinical services in primary treatment options, sexual health, exercise, nutrition, androgen deprivation therapy, pelvic floor physiotherapy, counseling services, and metastatic disease management.[61]

What strategies or rituals do you practice for preventing burnout or empathy fatigue?
That is a very good question! I usually make sure to take time off and not overbook myself. I also like to add movements into my day, for example, move my shoulders, back, or neck between sessions, because at times I may be so involved with someone's story that I forget to move and become very stiff. Mindfulness and meditation during sessions also help ground myself. After I leave work I tend to walk home and visualize distancing myself from work as best as possible and I also like to incorporate a movement ritual to symbolize this distancing through physically "moving the energy" around the room. What I think helps

---

59   (BC Cancer, n.d.)
60   (Statista, n.d.)
61   (Prostate Cancer Supportive Care, n.d.)

me the most to avoid burnout or fatigue is that I believe that the work that we do at PCSC and the mental health support that I can give to patients are making a positive impact in prostate cancer survivors' lives, and for that I am grateful.

Any other comments?
I feel that being diagnosed with cancer can have a lot of impact on someone's emotions. We can feel devastated, sad, angry, etc., but in my experience I have also seen it create opportunities for patients to re-evaluate their life and the lives of others around them. Cancer diagnosis or living with cancer may offer a chance for survivors to foster compassion and forgiveness, value relationships, prioritize what really is important, and maybe learn to become more adaptable and fluid.

The Prostate Cancer Supportive Care is a program funded by BC provincial health organizations and private donations—partnered with the University of British Columbia, the Vancouver General Hospital, the University of British Columbia Foundation, and Vancouver Coastal Health.[62] For more information visit https://pcscprogram.ca.

Physiotherapy

Physiotherapists have been identified both as key workers to bridge the gap between physical and mental health, and as essential team members to multidisciplinary care for management of distorted body imaging and anxiety disorders.[63] Additionally, by promoting physical activity and exercise, physiotherapists can improve patients' physical and mental health and increase social interactions, which can increase their overall sense of wellbeing.[64]

As mentioned in Chapter 8, strength training and aerobic exercise improve prostate cancer-specific anxiety, perceived stress, social support, self-efficacy, and self-esteem in prostate cancer survivors.[65, 66] Other benefits of exercise, such as improving sleep, increasing libido, increasing energy and stamina, increasing mental alertness, and improving endurance, can have a positive effect on mental health status.[67] The physiological changes from exercise affecting psychological health can be attributed to increasing blood supply to the brain and optimizing the hypothalamic–pituitary–adrenal (HPA) axis, which mediates the effect of stress.[68]

---

62 (Prostate Cancer Supportive Care, n.d.)
63 (Heywood *et al.*, 2022)
64 (Guszkowska, 2004)
65 (Chung *et al.*, 2022)
66 (Kang *et al.*, 2022)
67 (Sharma *et al.*, 2006)
68 (Guszkowska, 2004)

Qigong, yoga therapy, and mindfulness

Alternative therapies such as qigong, yoga, and mindfulness may play a role in improving prostate cancer distress and psychological symptoms. Over 50 percent of cancer patients in Australia and in the United States seek a "holistic" option or complementary medicine as adjunct to standard medical cancer care.[69]

Medical qigong, a mind–body practice, which is part of the traditional Chinese medicine practice, may have significant psychological benefits in cancer patients—including reduced tension, anxiety, depression, and fatigue.[70] Additionally, qigong seems to increase heart rate variability, therefore having a positive effect on autonomic dysfunction, which has been linked to improving psychological health status.[71]

Yoga is an ancient Indian philosophy that integrates practices of inner awareness, breathing, and body movement or postures. Therapeutic yoga adapts these practices for health related benefits, and in cancer care commonly involves physical postures, breathing, and meditation.[72] A mixed-practice yoga therapy program, combining mindful breathing, poses, and stretches seems to be effective in improving cancer-related fatigue in patients undergoing radiation therapy and/or chemotherapy.[73] Yoga therapy may also be feasible to be performed before prostatectomy surgery and may have positive quality-of-life outcomes such as increased physical and social wellbeing.[74] Additionally, a combination of gentle yoga and mindfulness meditation may improve prostate cancer survivors, spiritual, social, and emotional wellbeing.[75]

Mindfulness is a self-regulatory *experience-oriented* meditative approach using sustained *non-judgemental* moment to moment awareness, fostering *curiosity, openness* and *acceptance*. There is good evidence supporting mindfulness in reducing anxiety, depression, fatigue, and perceived stress in the cancer population.[76] More specifically, a feasibility pilot study demonstrated that a stress reduction mindfulness program improved the anxiety and fear of prostate cancer patients on active surveillance, and increased post-traumatic growth (re-evaluation and profound transformation of one's life outlook).[77]

Heart rate variability biofeedback (HRVB)

Biofeedback uses audiovisual cuing from information coming from electrical sensors connected to the patient for the purpose of improving body awareness

69 (Oh *et al.*, 2010)
70 (Oh *et al.*, 2010)
71 (Lee *et al.*, 2022)
72 (Song *et al.*, 2021)
73 (Song *et al.*, 2021)
74 (Kaushik *et al.*, 2021)
75 (Bryan *et al.*, 2021)
76 (Marinovic & Hunter, 2022)
77 (Victorson *et al.*, 2017)

and promoting functional changes. Most cancer studies combining HRVB with paced breathing to stimulate parasympathetic tone and increase heart rate variability showed a trend of improving pain levels, depression, anxiety, sleep disturbances, and cognitive performance.[78] Implementation of a home-based HRVB program may improve these psychological effects; however, it may not be accessible to every cancer patient as the most reliable devices can be very costly. HeartMath emWave seems to be the most common software and device used in cancer research for HRVB.[79]

PSYCHOLOGICAL HEALTH FOR CANCER HEALTH PROFESSIONALS

The dynamic, challenging, emotionally demanding, time sensitive, and stressful field of oncology may particularly challenge healthcare workers' psychological health status. Approximately one-third of oncologists, oncology nurses, and psychosocial therapists working in cancer care have reported symptoms of *burnout*, including high emotional exhaustion, high depersonalization, and low personal accomplishment.[80] Oncology workers may also be at increased risk for *compassion fatigue*, which is defined as repeated traumatic stress combined with burnout, and has been linked to anxiety, stress, and decreased job/career satisfaction, affecting work and home environments.[81] Recent scholars have suggested that *empathy fatigue* or *empathy distress* may be a more appropriate term than compassion fatigue as, contrasting with compassion, empathy may provoke negative affect feelings.[82] Symptoms associated with empathy distress (compassion fatigue) may include: increased negative emotions, intrusive thoughts, difficulty separating work from life, lowered tolerance, increased outbursts of anger, hypervigilance, depression, decreased work enjoyment, decreased feeling of work competence, and loss of hope.[83] *Grief* from losing a patient, or from difficult medical knowledge about the patient, may promote feelings of powerlessness, self-doubt, guilt, shame, and failure in oncology professionals.[84] Grief may also stem partially from health professionals' sense of responsibility towards their patients' lives, and its symptoms may last for hours without entirely disappearing.[85] When grief is not addressed or treated, it may result in health professionals feeling less compassionate toward their patients, leading to compassion fatigue.[86] Certain grief avoidance strategies—such as compartmentalization and

---

78 (Spada *et al.*, 2022)
79 (Spada *et al.*, 2022)
80 (Granek & Nakash, 2022)
81 (Pérez-García *et al.*, 2021)
82 (Seppälä *et al.*, 2017)
83 (Figley, 2002)
84 (Granek *et al.*, 2012)
85 (Laor-Maayany *et al.*, 2020)
86 (Laor-Maayany *et al.*, 2020)

emotional and physical distancing from patients—may impact health providers' quality of care, therapeutic decision making, and patient outcome.[87]

Managing emotions such as grief and implementing efficacious strategies to reduce empathy distress and burnout should be a priority in oncology practices. These methods and strategies may empower oncology workers with sufficient emotional resilience and confidence for delivering improved *client-focused* care.

Developing emotional resilience through self-caring

How can self-caring improve psychological resilience and prevent burnout or empathy fatigue in oncology care? A few studies have demonstrated the importance of engaging in routine self-caring practices, including mindfulness, grounding techniques, good sleep hygiene, gratitude practices, self-compassion, and emotional awareness, in reducing physiotherapists and oncology workers' clinical stress, anxiety, and emotional distress.[88, 89] Managing health workers' emotional health became even more important after the COVID-19 pandemic, as fear and uncertainty heightened their mental distress.[90] The basis of self-caring is fundamental for compassionate care, as health professionals need to be emotionally "fit" to be able to be fully present for others. The analogy of having to put on the oxygen mask first in a plane emergency before helping others illustrates the importance of self-caring.

There seems to be an increased demand all over the world for healthcare workers' psychosocial support initiatives in hospitals and health clinics, especially since the pandemic.[91, 92] One example is the introduction of a cognitive fitness program and mental health support counseling services at the Hospital for Special Surgery (NY) and NYU's Rusk Rehabilitation (USA) for their staff, including physiotherapists.[93] Another example is the development of CREATE (Compassion, REsilience And TEambuilding) at the Princess Margaret Cancer Centre in Toronto, Canada, which is a psychosocial intervention delivered to multidisciplinary frontline and oncology teams.[94]

There are many modes of burnout and empathy fatigue prevention practices. The most common ones highlighted in the literature include self-compassion training, mindfulness, yoga, compassion fatigue resiliency, and physical activity.

---

87   (Granek *et al.*, 2012)
88   (Klawonn *et al.*, 2019)
89   (Pfaff *et al.*, 2017)
90   (Datta *et al.*, 2020)
91   (Castillo-Sánchez *et al.*, 2022)
92   (Alexopoulos *et al.*, 2022)
93   (Wojciechowski, 2022)
94   (Shapiro *et al.*, 2021)

Self-compassion training

Self-compassion as defined by Neff has three key elements: self-kindness, common humanity, and mindfulness.[95] Nurturing self-compassion by enhancing the understanding that being mortal, imperfect, and vulnerable is part of the human experience[96] may foster kindness and forgiveness towards oneself.[97] Self-compassion skills (different from self-care) can be practiced on the job when pain or suffering arises, and may offer oncology workers greater work engagement, less emotional and physical exhaustion, greater professional life satisfaction, lower levels of burnout, and improved mental resilience.[98] *Compassion with equanimity* practice is a good example of self-compassion practice that can be easily integrated during patient interaction to remind providers that they are not fully in control of the outcome. During this practice, upon in-breath, providers imagine they are bringing in compassion, kindness, and emotional support for themselves, recognizing stress and empathic pain created during patient interaction. During out-breath, providers emanate compassion towards patients, validating their suffering, and identifying their own concern towards patients' wellbeing.[99] Other practices developed by Neff and Fingley include supportive touch (using breathing and hand touching of the heart to produce a parasympathetic response) and self-talking the three concepts of self-compassion during stressful situations.[100] The website self-compassion.org also provides a list of self-compassion exercises and guided practices for free.

Accelerated Recovery Program (ARP)

The ARP is a five-session model developed by Gentry, Baranowsky, and Dunning.[101] This program was designed for a variety of professionals working in a demanding and stressful workplace, with the goal to minimize or prevent symptoms associated with empathy distress (compassion fatigue (CF)). Goals of this program include recognizing symptoms and triggers of CF, identifying resources and strategies to reduce CF, learning grounding techniques, mastering arousal reduction methods, and implementing a supportive aftercare plan. The elements covered in the ARP are:

- Fostering therapeutic alliance
- Quantifying and qualifying symptoms of CF
- Learning anxiety reduction tools
- Improving the narrative of self-awareness, exposure and resolution of secondary traumatic stress

---

95 (Neff, 2003)
96 (Neff, n.d.)
97 (Kotera & Van Gordon, 2021)
98 (Neff et al., 2020)
99 (Neff et al., 2020)
100 (Neff et al., 2020)
101 (Gentry et al., 2002)

- Changing negative beliefs through cognitive restructuring and incorporating PATHWAYS, which is the aftercare resiliency model.[102]

A similar compassion-fatigue resiliency program implemented for six weeks in a regional cancer center demonstrated a reduction in oncology workers' perceived level of stress, by increasing awareness of CF symptoms and adopting self-care resiliency practices.[103]

Yoga

Yoga practices may offer a guiding path for physiotherapists and oncology workers to enhance self-compassion and self-love.[104] Yoga therapy, as a mind–body intervention approach, may improve healthcare professionals' stress levels, burnout, and sleep quality.[105]

A five-week program of yoga and whole-person biopsychosocial–spiritual model classes (composed of 60-minute weekly sessions incorporating education, mindful movements, meditation, and breathing practices) showed improvements in perceived stress and anxiety, self-compassion, mindfulness, and depression in graduate healthcare students (after 10 weeks). Each week, classes were focused on one of the five yoga *koshas,* which in yoga philosophy represents the human being's physical, intellectual, psychosocial, energetical, and spiritual layers.[106] This may be a short, practical, and acceptable program for fast-paced and demanding working environments such as oncology practices, which can potentially improve healthcare workers' short-term symptoms of CF. However, its feasibility and acceptability still need to be tested in cancer care, including in prostate cancer clinics and hospital settings.

Mindfulness

As defined by Kabat-Zinn, mindfulness is "the awareness that emerges through paying attention on purpose, in the present moment, and nonjudgmentally to the unfolding of experience moment by moment."[107] According to Kabat-Zinn, mindfulness practices may help to cultivate qualities such as patience, trust, and acceptance, which can contribute to self-compassion.[108] Mindfulness practices have shown to be effective for self-managing healthcare professionals' occupationally-related stress and improving their sense of wellbeing.[109]

The mindfulness-based stress reduction program (MBSR) developed by Kabat-Zinn has become a model for other mindfulness programs in health

102 (Figley, 2002)
103 (Pfaff *et al.*, 2017)
104 (Prosko, 2019)
105 (Di Mario *et al.*, 2023)
106 (Klawonn *et al.*, 2019)
107 (Kabat-Zinn, 2003)
108 (Poulin *et al.*, 2008)
109 (Di Mario *et al.*, 2023)

research, and includes: standardized weekly classes led by an instructor with mindfulness training (usually 6 weeks), daily 45-minute practices assigned each week, and a day of mindfulness meditation usually at the end of the program. These classes may start with a brief relaxation and breathing exercise before the content is presented, ending with a quote or theme for personal reflection.[110]

GROUNDING RITUALS DURING CLINICAL PRACTICE

Grounding techniques or rituals can be used in clinical practice (during and after interactions with patients) to help physiotherapists and oncology clinicians reset, find their body, be present, or obtain emotional balance. The concept of grounding in psychotherapy was originated by Alexander Lowen, and was based on the concept that emotional wellness is achieved by physically, mentally, and energetically connecting to the earth.[111] Grounding can also be described as individuals' ability to be present with their body and mind in the present moment, for example, feeling their feet on the ground while paying attention to their breathing.

Grounding rituals can be used during or after therapeutic sessions. For example, as suggested by Prosko,[112] hand washing can be used as a ritual time, where clinicians acknowledge the end of a session before the beginning of another. Clinicians can focus on the sensation of warm water falling onto the skin, while using a forceful exhale to represent the end of the clinical interaction with the previous patient.

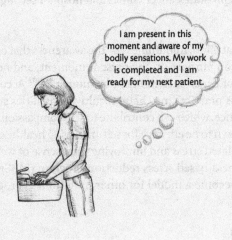

I am present in this moment and aware of my bodily sensations. My work is completed and I am ready for my next patient.

110 (Pérez *et al.*, 2022)
111 (de Tord & Bräuninger, 2015)
112 (Prosko, 2019)

PAIN CATEGORIZATION AND THE ROLE OF PSYCHOSOCIAL FACTORS

As mentioned in Chapter 4, pain is a physical and *emotional* experience that can be influenced by psychosocial factors.[113] Pain is highly prevalent in prostate cancer survivors[114] and is associated with fatigue, depression and anxiety.[115] Cancer-related distress, for example, hyperarousal and intrusion, can have an influence on pain, therefore psychosocial interventions such as CBT or other stress management psychotherapy may have an important role in managing cancer pain.[116]

Other factors to consider when treating cancer pain are determining classification and mechanisms of pain, as well as their emotional response towards pain. In addition to administering psychosocial questionnaires mentioned for screening anxiety, depression, and stress, other pain questionnaires, such as the Central Sensitization Inventory (CSI), the Pain Catastrophizing Scale (PCS), and the Leeds Assessment of Neuropathic Symptoms and Signs (LANSS), may be useful to improve clinicians' understanding of prostate cancer survivors' pain mechanism and influences. The CSI has a part A and a part B; a score of over 40 on part A has been shown to be valid and reliable for determining central sensitization.[117] The PCS has three subtypes—rumination, helplessness, and magnification—which have been correlated to pain catastrophization or increased pain-related negative thought, emotional distress, and increased pain. A PCS score of 30 represents clinically significant levels of catastrophizing.[118] The LANSS is a questionnaire combined with examination items validated for identifying neuropathic pain.[119]

113 (International Association for the Study of Pain, n.d.)
114 (van den Beuken-van Everdingen *et al.*, 2007)
115 (Walsh *et al.*, 2022)
116 (Walsh *et al.*, 2022)
117 (Neblett *et al.*, 2015)
118 (Sullivan *et al.*, 1995)
119 (Bennett, 2001)

Age:_____   Sex: M(_____)   F(_____)

Everyone experiences painful situations at some point in their lives. Such experiences may include headaches, tooth pain, joint or muscle pain. People are often exposed to situations that may cause pain, such as illness, injury, dental procedures or surgery.

We are interested in the types of thoughts and feelings that you have when you are in pain. Listed below are thirteen statements describing different thoughts and feelings that may be associated with pain. Using the following scale, please indicate the degree to which you have these thoughts and feelings when you are experiencing pain.

0 – not at all   1 – to a slight degree   2 – to a moderate degree   3 – to a great degree   4 – all the time

---

When I'm in pain...

1   ☐   I worry all the time about whether the pain will end.

2   ☐   I feel I can't go on.

3   ☐   It's terrible and I think it's never going to get any better.

4   ☐   It's awful and I feel that it overwhelms me.

5   ☐   I feel I can't stand it anymore.

6   ☐   I become afraid that the pain will get worse.

7   ☐   I keep thinking of other painful events.

8   ☐   I anxiously want the pain to go away.

9   ☐   I can't seem to keep it out of my mind.

10 ☐   I keep thinking about how much it hurts.

11 ☐   I keep thinking about how badly I want the pain to stop.

12 ☐   There's nothing I can do to reduce the intensity of the pain.

13 ☐   I wonder whether something serious may happen.

...Total

PCS - United Kingdom/English - Version of 28 Feb 17 - Mapi.
ID057817 / PCS_AU1.0_eng-GB.doc

FIGURE 9.3: PAIN CATASTROPHIZING SCALE (PCS)
Copyright © Pain Catastrophizing Scale (PCS)

CENTRAL SENSITIZATION INVENTORY: PART A

Name: _____   Date: _____

Please circle the best response to the right of each statement.

1	I feel tired and unrefreshed when I wake from sleeping.	Never	Rarely	Sometimes	Often	Always
2	My muscles feel stiff and achy.	Never	Rarely	Sometimes	Often	Always
3	I have anxiety attacks.	Never	Rarely	Sometimes	Often	Always
4	I grind or clench my teeth.	Never	Rarely	Sometimes	Often	Always
5	I have problems with diarrhea and/or constipation.	Never	Rarely	Sometimes	Often	Always
6	I need help in performing my daily activities.	Never	Rarely	Sometimes	Often	Always
7	I am sensitive to bright lights.	Never	Rarely	Sometimes	Often	Always
8	I get tired very easily when I am physically active.	Never	Rarely	Sometimes	Often	Always
9	I feel pain all over my body.	Never	Rarely	Sometimes	Often	Always
10	I have headaches.	Never	Rarely	Sometimes	Often	Always
11	I feel discomfort in my bladder and/or burning when I urinate.	Never	Rarely	Sometimes	Often	Always
12	I do not sleep well.	Never	Rarely	Sometimes	Often	Always
13	I have difficulty concentrating.	Never	Rarely	Sometimes	Often	Always
14	I have skin problems such as dryness, itchiness, or rashes.	Never	Rarely	Sometimes	Often	Always
15	Stress makes my physical symptoms get worse.	Never	Rarely	Sometimes	Often	Always
16	I feel sad or depressed.	Never	Rarely	Sometimes	Often	Always
17	I have low energy.	Never	Rarely	Sometimes	Often	Always
18	I have muscle tension in my neck and shoulders.	Never	Rarely	Sometimes	Often	Always
19	I have pain in my jaw.	Never	Rarely	Sometimes	Often	Always
20	Certain smells, such as perfumes, make me feel dizzy and nauseated.	Never	Rarely	Sometimes	Often	Always
21	I have to urinate frequently.	Never	Rarely	Sometimes	Often	Always
22	My legs feel uncomfortable and restless when I am trying to go to sleep at night.	Never	Rarely	Sometimes	Often	Always
23	I have difficulty remembering things.	Never	Rarely	Sometimes	Often	Always
24	I suffered trauma as a child.	Never	Rarely	Sometimes	Often	Always
25	I have pain in my pelvic area.	Never	Rarely	Sometimes	Often	Always

Total=

Rev. 6-3-2015

FIGURE 9.4A: CENTRAL SENSITIZATION INVENTORY (CSI)

This scale is in the public domain. For download in all available languages; visit: www.pridedallas.com/questionnaires

CENTRAL SENSITIZATION INVENTORY: PART B

Name: _____   Date: _____

Have you been diagnosed by a doctor with any of the following disorders?

Please check the box to the right for each diagnosis and write the year of the diagnosis.

		NO	YES	Year Diagnosed
1	Restless Leg Syndrome			
2	Chronic Fatigue Syndrome			
3	Fibromyalgia			
4	Temporomandibular Joint Disorder (TMJ)			
5	Migraine or tension headaches			
6	Irritable Bowel Syndrome			
7	Multiple Chemical Sensitivities			
8	Neck Injury (including whiplash)			
9	Anxiety or Panic Attacks			
10	Depression			

Rev. 6-3-2015

FIGURE 9.4B: CENTRAL SENSITIZATION INVENTORY (CSI)[120]

This scale is in the public domain. For download in all available languages; visit: www.pridedallas.com/questionnaires

---

120 (Mayer *et al.*, 2012)

CONCLUSION

This chapter presented the importance for well-equipping physiotherapists and oncology healthcare professionals with understanding the signs and symptoms of mental health issues and the process of how to provide appropriate support and resources for those in need. Prostate cancer survivors may strongly benefit from psychological screening and psychosocial interventions, as they are at higher risks for mental distress, which can negatively affect their symptoms, prognosis, and quality of life. Additionally, building a strong therapeutic relationship between patients and clinicians can improve patients' outcomes and promote better overall health and wellbeing. Compassionate listening and caring can go a long way in helping prostate cancer patients feel validated and heard, which can ultimately lead to more positive psychological responses and health outcomes. Self-compassion resilience training, yoga therapy, or mindfulness practices may aid cancer health workers to reduce or prevent occupational-related stress, burnout, and compassion fatigue. Therefore, it may be highly beneficial for cancer health professionals to practice mindfulness, mind–body routines, or attend formal stress reduction programs in order to improve their psychological resilience, job satisfaction, and wellbeing. It may also be of value for healthcare graduate students to deepen their knowledge of mental health and self-caring practices during their training years for improving overall competency, confidence, safety, and wellness in the workplace.

REFERENCES

Alexopoulos, P., Roukas, D., Efkarpidis, A., Konstantopoulou, G., et al. (2022). Hospital workforce mental reaction to the pandemic in a low COVID-19 burden setting: A cross-sectional clinical study. European Archives of Psychiatry and Clinical Neuroscience, 272(1), 95–105. https://doi.org/10.1007/s00406-021-01262-y

Avery, K., Donovan, J., Peters, T.J., Shaw, C., Gotoh, M., & Abrams, P. (2004). ICIQ: A brief and robust measure for evaluating the symptoms and impact of urinary incontinence. Neurourology and Urodynamics, 23(4), 322–330. https://doi.org/10.1002/nau.20041

BC Cancer (n.d.). Cancer incidence, British Colombia, by cancer type, age at diagnosis and sex. Retrieved April 3, 2023, from https://bccandataanalytics.shinyapps.io/IncidenceCounts

Bedretdinova, D., Fritel, X., Zins, M., & Ringa, V. (2016). The effect of urinary incontinence on health-related quality of life: Is it similar in men and women? Urology, 91, 83–89. https://doi.org/10.1016/j.urology.2015.12.034

Bennett, M. (2001). The LANSS Pain Scale: The Leeds assessment of neuropathic symptoms and signs. Pain, 92(1–2), 147–157. https://doi.org/10.1016/s0304-3959(00)00482-6

Bowie, J., Brunckhorst, O., Stewart, R., Dasgupta, P., & Ahmed, K. (2022). Body image, self-esteem, and sense of masculinity in patients with prostate cancer: A qualitative meta-synthesis. Journal of Cancer Survivorship, 16(1), 95–110. https://doi.org/10.1007/s11764-021-01007-9

Bryan, S., Zipp, G., & Breitkreuz, D. (2021). The effects of mindfulness meditation and gentle yoga on spiritual well-being in cancer survivors: A pilot study. Alternative Therapies in Health and Medicine, 27(3), 32–38.

Castillo-Sánchez, G., Sacristán-Martín, O., Hernández, M.A., Muñoz, I., de la Torre, I., & Franco-Martín, M. (2022). Online mindfulness experience for emotional support to healthcare staff in times of Covid-19. *Journal of Medical Systems, 46*(3), 1–11. https://doi.org/10.1007/s10916-022-01799-y

Center for Epidemiologic Studies Depression Scale (CESD). (2017, April 7). CESD-R. Retrieved on September 25, 2023, from https://cesd-r.com/about-cesdr

Chambers, S.K., Zajdlewicz, L., Youlden, D.R., Holland, J.C., & Dunn, J. (2014). The validity of the distress thermometer in prostate cancer populations. *Psycho-Oncology, 23*(2), 195–203. https://doi.org/10.1002/pon.3391

Chiang, Y.-C., Couper, J., Chen, J.-W., Lin, K.-J., & Wu, H.-P. (2022). Predictive value of the Distress Thermometer score for risk of suicide in patients with cancer. *Supportive Care in Cancer, 30*(6), 5047–5053. https://doi.org/10.1007/s00520-022-06801-4

Chien, C.-H., Liu, K.-L., Chien, H.-T., & Liu, H.-E. (2014). The effects of psychosocial strategies on anxiety and depression of patients diagnosed with prostate cancer: A systematic review. *International Journal of Nursing Studies, 51*(1), 28–38. https://doi.org/10.1016/j.ijnurstu.2012.12.019

Chung, K.H., Park, S.B., Streckmann, F., Wiskemann, J., *et al.* (2022). Mechanisms, mediators, and moderators of the effects of exercise on chemotherapy-induced peripheral neuropathy. *Cancers, 14*(5), Article 5. https://doi.org/10.3390/cancers14051224

College of Physical Therapists of British Columbia (CPTBC) (2023). Clients at risk. Retrieved September 21, 2023 from https://cptbc.org/physical-therapists/practice-resources/advice-to-consider/clients-at-risk

College of Physiotherapists of Alberta (n.d.). Good practice: When a patient expresses suicidal ideation. Retrieved March 6, 2023, from www.cpta.ab.ca/news-and-updates/news/good-practice-when-a-patient-expresses-suicidal-ideation

College of Physiotherapists of Ontario (n.d.). Strategies to support patients at risk. Retrieved March 6, 2023, from www.collegept.org/registrants/pt-resources/patient-support-strategies

Costanzo, E.S., Sood, A.K., & Lutgendorf, S.K. (2011). Biobehavioral influences on cancer progression. *Immunology and Allergy Clinics, 31*(1), 109–132. https://doi.org/10.1016/j.iac.2010.09.001

Cuypers, M., Lamers, R.E.D., Kil, P.J.M., Cornel, E.B., van de Poll-Franse, L.V., & de Vries, M. (2018). The impact of prostate cancer diagnosis and treatment decision-making on health-related quality of life before treatment onset. *Supportive Care in Cancer, 26*(4), 1297–1304. https://doi.org/10.1007/s00520-017-3953-8

Datta, S.S., Mukherjee, A., Ghose, S., Bhattacharya, S., & Gyawali, B. (2020). Addressing the mental health challenges of cancer care workers in LMICs during the time of the COVID-19 pandemic. *JCO Global Oncology, 6*, 1490–1493. https://doi.org/10.1200/GO.20.00470

de Tord, P., & Bräuninger, I. (2015). Grounding: Theoretical application and practice in dance movement therapy. *The Arts in Psychotherapy, 43*, 16–22. https://doi.org/10.1016/j.aip.2015.02.001

Di Mario, S., Cocchiara, R.A., & La Torre, G. (2023). The use of yoga and mindfulness-based interventions to reduce stress and burnout in healthcare workers: An umbrella review. *Alternative Therapies in Health and Medicine, 29*(1), 29–35.

Dinesh, A., Pinto, S.H.P., Brunckhorst, O., Dasgupta, P., & Ahmed, K. (2021). Anxiety, depression and urological cancer outcomes: A systematic review. *Urologic Oncology: Seminars and Original Investigations, 39*(12), 816–828. https://doi.org/10.1016/j.urolonc.2021.08.003

Esser, P., Hartung, T.J., Friedrich, M., Johansen, C., *et al.* (2018). The Generalized Anxiety Disorder Screener (GAD-7) and the anxiety module of the Hospital and Depression Scale (HADS-A) as screening tools for generalized anxiety disorder among cancer patients. *Psycho-Oncology, 27*(6), 1509–1516. https://doi.org/10.1002/pon.4681

Felde, G., Ebbesen, M.H., & Hunskaar, S. (2017). Anxiety and depression associated with urinary incontinence: A 10-year follow-up study from the Norwegian HUNT study (EPINCONT). *Neurourology and Urodynamics, 36*(2), 322–328. https://doi.org/10.1002/nau.22921

Fervaha, G., Izard, J.P., Tripp, D.A., Aghel, N., *et al.* (2020). Psychological morbidity associated with prostate cancer: Rates and predictors of depression in the RADICAL PC study. *Canadian Urological Association Journal, 15*(6). https://doi.org/10.5489/cuaj.6912

Figley, C.R. (Ed.). (2002). *Treating Compassion Fatigue* (1st ed.). Routledge. https://doi.org/10.4324/9780203890318

Fuertes, J.N., Mislowack, A., Bennett, J., Paul, L., Gilbert, T.C., Fontan, G., & Boylan, L.S. (2007). The physician–patient working alliance. *Patient Education and Counseling, 66*(1), 29–36. https://doi.org/10.1016/j.pec.2006.09.013

Gentry, E., Baranowski, A., & Dunning, K. (2002). ARP: The Accelerated Recovery Program (ARP) for Compassion Fatigue. In C. Fingley (ed.), *Treating Compassion Fatigue, 1st edition.* Abingdon: Brunner-Routledge.

Granek, L., & Nakash, O. (2022). Oncology healthcare professionals' mental health during the COVID-19 pandemic. *Current Oncology, 29*(6), 4054–4067. https://doi.org/10.3390/curroncol29060323

Granek, L., Tozer, R., Mazzotta, P., Ramjaun, A., & Krzyzanowska, M. (2012). Nature and impact of grief over patient loss on oncologists' personal and professional lives. *Archives of Internal Medicine, 172*(12), 964–966. https://doi.org/10.1001/archinternmed.2012.1426

Guszkowska, M. (2004). [Effects of exercise on anxiety, depression and mood]. *Psychiatria Polska, 38*(4), 611–620.

Heywood, S.E., Connaughton, J., Kinsella, R., Black, S., Bicchi, N., & Setchell, J. (2022). Physical therapy and mental health: A scoping review. *Physical Therapy, 102*(11), pzac102. https://doi.org/10.1093/ptj/pzac102

ICIQ (n.d.). International Consultation on Incontinence Questionnaire–Urinary Incontinence Short Form (ICIQ-UI-SF). Retrieved May 1, 2023, from https://iciq.net/iciq-ui-sf

International Association for the Study of Pain. (n.d.). Terminology. Retrieved February 13, 2023, from www.iasp-pain.org/resources/terminology/

Jacobsen, P.B., & Jim, H.S. (2008). Psychosocial interventions for anxiety and depression in adult cancer patients: Achievements and challenges. *CA: A Cancer Journal for Clinicians, 58*(4), 214–230. https://doi.org/10.3322/CA.2008.0003

Kabat-Zinn, J. (2003). Mindfulness-based interventions in context: Past, present, and future. *Clinical Psychology: Science & Practice, 10*(2), 144–156. https://doi.org/10.1093/clipsy.bpg016

Kang, D.-W., Fairey, A.S., Boulé, N.G., Field, C.J., Wharton, S.A., & Courneya, K.S. (2022). A randomized trial of the effects of exercise on anxiety, fear of cancer progression and quality of life in prostate cancer patients on active surveillance. *Journal of Urology, 207*(4), 814–822. https://doi.org/10.1097/JU.0000000000002334

Kaushik, D., Shah, P., Mukherjee, N., Ji, N., *et al.* (2021). LBA02-03 A phase II randomized clinical trial of yoga in men with prostate cancer. *Journal of Urology, 206*(Supplement 3). https://doi.org/10.1097/JU.0000000000002149.03

Klawonn, A., Kernan, D., & Lynskey, J. (2019). A 5-week seminar on the biopsychosocial-spiritual model of self-care improves anxiety, self-compassion, mindfulness, depression, and stress in graduate healthcare students. *International Journal of Yoga Therapy, 29*(1), 81–89. https://doi.org/10.17761/D-18-2019-00026

Kleiner, M.J., Kinsella, E.A., Miciak, M., Teachman, G., McCabe, E., & Walton, D.M. (2021). An integrative review of the qualities of a "good" physiotherapist. *Physiotherapy Theory and Practice, 39*(1), 1–28. https://doi.org/10.1080/09593985.2021.1999354

Kotera, Y., & Van Gordon, W. (2021). Effects of self-compassion training on work-related well-being: A systematic review. *Frontiers in Psychology, 12.* www.frontiersin.org/articles/10.3389/fpsyg.2021.630798

Kroenke, K., Spitzer, R.L., & Williams, J.B. (2001). The PHQ-9: Validity of a brief depression severity measure. *Journal of General Internal Medicine, 16*(9), 606–613. https://doi.org/10.1046/j.1525-1497.2001.016009606.x

Lai, H.H., Rawal, A., Shen, B., & Vetter, J. (2016). The relationship between anxiety and overactive bladder or urinary incontinence symptoms in the clinical population. *Urology, 98*, 50–57. https://doi.org/10.1016/j.urology.2016.07.013

Laor-Maayany, R., Goldzweig, G., Hasson-Ohayon, I., Bar-Sela, G., Engler-Gross, A., & Braun, M. (2020). Compassion fatigue among oncologists: The role of grief, sense of failure, and exposure to suffering and death. *Supportive Care in Cancer, 28*(4), 2025–2031. https://doi.org/10.1007/s00520-019-05009-3

Lee, Y.-H., Chang, Y.-P., Lee, J.-T., Lee, D.-C., Huang, E.-Y., & Lai, L.-J.T. (2022). Heart rate variability as an indicator of the beneficial effects of Qigong and mindfulness training on the mind-body well-being of cancer survivors. *Supportive Care in Cancer, 31*(1), 59. https://doi.org/10.1007/s00520-022-07476-7

Levine, G.N., Cohen, B.E., Commodore-Mensah, Y., Fleury, J., et al. (2021). Psychological health, well-being, and the mind-heart-body connection: A scientific statement from the American Heart Association. *Circulation, 143*(10), e763–e783. https://doi.org/10.1161/CIR.0000000000000947

Majerova, K., Zvarik, M., Ricon-Becker, I., Hanalis-Miller, T., et al. (2022). Increased sympathetic modulation in breast cancer survivors determined by measurement of heart rate variability. *Scientific Reports, 12*(1), Article 1. https://doi.org/10.1038/s41598-022-18865-7

Marinovic, D.A., & Hunter, R.L. (2022). Examining the interrelationships between mindfulness-based interventions, depression, inflammation, and cancer survival. *CA: A Cancer Journal for Clinicians, 72*(5), 490–502. https://doi.org/10.3322/caac.21733

Mayer, T.G., Neblett, R., Cohen, H., Howard, K.J., et al. (2012). The development and psychometric validation of the Central Sensitization Inventory (CSI). *Pain Practice, 12*(4), 276–285. https://doi.org/10.1111/j.1533-2500.2011.00493.x

McConkey, R.W. (2016). The psychosocial dimensions of fatigue in men treated for prostate cancer. *International Journal of Urological Nursing, 10*(1), 37–43. https://doi.org/10.1111/ijun.12089

McKernan, L.C., Walsh, C.G., Reynolds, W.S., Crofford, L.J., Dmochowski, R.R., & Williams, D.A. (2018). Psychosocial co-morbidities in Interstitial Cystitis/Bladder Pain Syndrome (IC/BPS): A systematic review. *Neurourology and Urodynamics, 37*(3), 926–941. https://doi.org/10.1002/nau.23421

National Cancer Institute (2014). Emotions and cancer. Retrieved September 20, 2023 from www.cancer.gov/about-cancer/coping/feelings

National Comprehensive Cancer Network (NCCN) (n.d.). Distress Thermometer Tool Translations. Retrieved March 6, 2023, from www.nccn.org/global/what-we-do/distress-thermometer-tool-translations

Neblett, R., Hartzell, M.M., Cohen, H., Mayer, T.G., Williams, M., Choi, Y., & Gatchel, R.J. (2015). Ability of the central sensitization inventory to identify central sensitivity syndromes in an outpatient chronic pain sample. *Clinical Journal of Pain, 31*(4), 323–332. https://doi.org/10.1097/AJP.0000000000000113

Neff, K. (n.d.). Definition and three elements of self compassion. Retrieved March 15, 2023, from https://self-compassion.org/the-three-elements-of-self-compassion-2

Neff, K.D. (2003). Self-compassion: An alternative conceptualization of a healthy attitude toward oneself. *Self and Identity, 2*(2), 85–101. https://doi.org/10.1080/15298860309032

Neff, K.D., Knox, M.C., Long, P., & Gregory, K. (2020). Caring for others without losing yourself: An adaptation of the Mindful Self-Compassion Program for healthcare communities. *Journal of Clinical Psychology, 76*(9), 1543–1562. https://doi.org/10.1002/jclp.23007

Oh, B., Butow, P., Mullan, B., Clarke, S., et al. (2010). Impact of Medical Qigong on quality of life, fatigue, mood and inflammation in cancer patients: A randomized controlled trial. *Annals of Oncology, 21*(3), 608–614. https://doi.org/10.1093/annonc/mdp479

Osório, F.L., Lima, M.P., & Chagas, M.H.N. (2015). Screening tools for psychiatry disorders in cancer setting: Caution when using. *Psychiatry Research, 229*(3), 739–742. https://doi.org/10.1016/j.psychres.2015.08.009

Pérez, V., Menéndez-Crispín, E.J., Sarabia-Cobo, C., de Lorena, P., Fernández-Rodríguez, A., & González-Vaca, J. (2022). Mindfulness-based intervention for the reduction of compassion fatigue and burnout in nurse caregivers of institutionalized older persons with dementia: A randomized controlled trial. *International Journal of Environmental Research and Public Health, 19*(18). https://doi.org/10.3390/ijerph191811441

Pérez-García, E., Ortega-Galán, Á.M., Ibáñez-Masero, O., Ramos-Pichardo, J.D., Fernández-Leyva, A., & Ruiz-Fernández, M.D. (2021). Qualitative study on the causes and consequences of compassion fatigue from the perspective of nurses. *International Journal of Mental Health Nursing, 30*(2), 469–478. https://doi.org/10.1111/inm.12807

Perry, S., McGrother, C.W., Turner, K., & Group, L.M.I.S. (2006). An investigation of the relationship between anxiety and depression and urge incontinence in women: Development of a psychological model. *British Journal of Health Psychology, 11*(3), 463–482. https://doi.org/10.1348/135910705X60742

Pfaff, K.A., Freeman-Gibb, L., Patrick, L.J., DiBiase, R., & Moretti, O. (2017). Reducing the "cost of caring" in cancer care: Evaluation of a pilot interprofessional compassion fatigue resiliency programme. *Journal of Interprofessional Care, 31*(4), 512–519. https://doi.org/10.1080/13561820.2017.1309364

Poulin, P.A., Mackenzie, C.S., Soloway, G., & Karayolas, E. (2008). Mindfulness training as an evidenced-based approach to reducing stress and promoting well-being among human services professionals. *International Journal of Health Promotion & Education, 46*(2), 72–80. https://doi.org/10.1080/14635240.2008.10708132

Prosko, S. (2019). Compassion in Pain Care. In N. Pearson, S. Prosko, & M. Sullivan (eds) *Yoga and Science in Pain Care: Treating the Person in Pain.* (pp.235–256). London: Singing Dragon Publishers.

Prostate Cancer Supportive Care (n.d.). About. Retrieved March 25, 2023, from https://pcscprogram.ca/pcsc-program/about

Saracino, R.M., Weinberger, M.I., Roth, A.J., Hurria, A., & Nelson, C.J. (2017). Assessing depression in a geriatric cancer population. *Psycho-Oncology, 26*(10), 1484–1490. https://doi.org/10.1002/pon.4160

Schnur, J.B., & Montgomery, G.H. (2010). A systematic review of therapeutic alliance, group cohesion, empathy, and goal consensus/collaboration in psychotherapeutic interventions in cancer: Uncommon factors? *Clinical Psychology Review, 30*(2), 238–247. https://doi.org/10.1016/j.cpr.2009.11.005

Seppälä, E.M., Simon-Thomas, E., Brown, S.L., Worline, M.C., Cameron, C.D., & Doty, J.R. (eds) (2017). *The Oxford Handbook of Compassion Science, 1st edition.* Oxford: Oxford University Press.

Shaffer, F., & Ginsberg, J.P. (2017). An overview of Heart Rate Variability metrics and norms. *Frontiers in Public Health, 5*, 258. https://doi.org/10.3389/fpubh.2017.00258

Shapiro, G.K., Psych, C., Schulz-Quach, C., Matthew, A., *et al.* (2021). *An Institutional Model for Health Care Workers' Mental Health During Covid-19. NEJM Catalyst – Innovations in Care Delivery, Commentary, 2*(2).

Sharma, A., Madaan, V., & Petty, F.D. (2006). Exercise for mental health. *Primary Care Companion to the Journal of Clinical Psychiatry, 8*(2), 106.

Smith, A.L., Leung, J., Kun, S., Zhang, R., *et al.* (2011). The effects of acute and chronic psychological stress on bladder function in a rodent model. *Urology, 78*(4), 967.e1-967.e7. https://doi.org/10.1016/j.urology.2011.06.041

Song, J., Wang, T., Wang, Y., Li, R., *et al.* (2021). The effectiveness of yoga on cancer-related fatigue: A systematic review and meta-analysis. *Oncology Nursing Forum, 48*(2), 207–228. https://doi.org/10.1188/21.ONF.207-228

Spada, G.E., Masiero, M., Pizzoli, S.F.M., & Pravettoni, G. (2022). Heart rate variability biofeedback in cancer patients: A scoping review. *Behavioral Sciences, 12*(10), Article 10. https://doi.org/10.3390/bs12100389

Statista (n.d.). British Columbia population by age and sex 2022. Retrieved April 3, 2023, from https://www.statista.com/statistics/605971/population-of-british-columbia-by-age-and-sex/

Sullivan, M.J.L., Bishop, S.R., & Pivik, J. (1995). The Pain Catastrophizing Scale: Development and validation. *Psychological Assessment, 7*(4), 524–532. https://doi.org/10.1037/1040-3590.7.4.524

Teunissen, D., Van Den Bosch, W., Van Weel, C., & Lagro-Janssen, T. (2006). "It can always happen": The impact of urinary incontinence on elderly men and women. *Scandinavian Journal of Primary Health Care, 24*(3), 166–173. https://doi.org/10.1080/02813430600739371

van den Beuken-van Everdingen, M.H.J., de Rijke, J.M., Kessels, A.G., Schouten, H.C., van Kleef, M., & Patijn, J. (2007). High prevalence of pain in patients with cancer in a large population-based study in The Netherlands. *Pain, 132*(3), 312–320. https://doi.org/10.1016/j.pain.2007.08.022

Victorson, D., Hankin, V., Burns, J., Weiland, R., *et al.* (2017). Feasibility, acceptability and preliminary psychological benefits of mindfulness meditation training in a sample of men diagnosed with prostate cancer on active surveillance: Results from a randomized controlled pilot trial. *Psycho-Oncology, 26*(8), 1155–1163. https://doi.org/10.1002/pon.4135

Wall, D., & Kristjanson, L. (2005). Men, culture and hegemonic masculinity: Understanding the experience of prostate cancer. *Nursing Inquiry, 12*(2), 87–97. https://doi.org/10.1111/j.1440-1800.2005.00258.x

Walsh, E.A., Pedreira, P.B., Moreno, P.I., Popok, P.J., *et al.* (2022). Pain, cancer-related distress, and physical and functional well-being among men with advanced prostate cancer. *Supportive Care in Cancer, 31*(1), 28–28. https://doi.org/10.1007/s00520-022-07453-0

Watkins, K.E., Eberhart, N., Hilton, L., Suttorp, M.J., Hepner, K.A., Clemens, J.Q., & Berry, S.H. (2011). Depressive disorders and panic attacks in women with bladder pain syndrome/interstitial cystitis: A population-based sample. *General Hospital Psychiatry, 33*(2), 143–149. https://doi.org/10.1016/j.genhosppsych.2011.01.004

Watts, S., Leydon, G., Birch, B., Prescott, P., Lai, L., Eardley, S., & Lewith, G. (2014). Depression and anxiety in prostate cancer: A systematic review and meta-analysis of prevalence rates. *BMJ Open, 4*(3), e003901. https://doi.org/10.1136/bmjopen-2013-003901

Wojciechowski, M. (2022). PTs and PTAs often tell patients to practice self-care: Now it's time for them to take their own advice. *APTA.org/APTA-Magazine*, July, 29–36.

World Health Organization (n.d.). Mental health. Retrieved February 27, 2023, from https://www.who.int/news-room/fact-sheets/detail/mental-health-strengthening-our-response

Yang, N., Xiao, H., Wang, W., Li, S., Yan, H., & Wang, Y. (2018). Effects of doctors' empathy abilities on the cellular immunity of patients with advanced prostate cancer treated by orchiectomy: The mediating role of patients' stigma, self-efficacy, and anxiety. *Patient Preference and Adherence, 12*, 1305–1314. https://doi.org/10.2147/PPA.S166460

Zorn, B.H., Montgomery, H., Pieper, K., Gray, M., & Steers, W.D. (1999). Urinary incontinence and depression. *Journal of Urology, 162*(1), 82–84. https://doi.org/10.1097/00005392-199907000-00020

CHAPTER 10

The Social Part 1: Sexual Health

Contributed by Dr. Jo Milios (men's health physiotherapist) PhD, MACP

INTRODUCTION

Sexuality, according to the (US) National Cancer Institute, refers to a person's behaviors, desires, and attitudes concerning sex and physical intimacy with others.[1] Male sexuality is influenced by various biological, psychological, and social factors that affect how men perceive and engage in sexual behavior. The

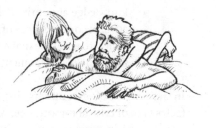

meaning of male sexuality is shaped by cultural, historical, and individual factors, and it can differ significantly among societies and individuals.[2] Some people argue that men often place significant emphasis on their genitals, particularly the penis, which is frequently regarded as the central physical aspect of masculinity.[3, 4] As a result, sexual health and penile changes become highly important topics in prostate cancer survivorship. After prostate cancer treatments, changes in sexual desire, erectile function, and penile length can have a profound impact on men's self-esteem, relationships, and overall sense of meaning in life.

This chapter, contributed by Dr. Jo Milios, PhD, will explore the topic of sexual health dysfunctions and treatment approaches within the context of prostate cancer care. It aims to provide a comprehensive and insightful analysis of the challenges and potential solutions related to sexual health issues that arise in individuals diagnosed with prostate cancer.

---

1   (National Cancer Institute, 2011)
2   (Tolman & Diamond, 2001)
3   (Danoff, 2011)
4   (Oswald et al., 2021)

SEXUAL HEALTH AND PROSTATE CANCER

As per the World Health Organization's (WHO) recommendations:

> Sexual health is fundamental to the overall health and wellbeing of individuals, couples and families, and to the social and economic development of communities and countries. Sexual health, when viewed affirmatively, requires a positive and respectful approach to sexuality and sexual relationships, as well as the possibility of having pleasurable and safe sexual experiences, free of coercion, discrimination and violence. The ability of men and women to achieve sexual health and wellbeing depends on their:
>
> - access to comprehensive, good-quality information about sex and sexuality;
> - knowledge about the risks they may face and their vulnerability to adverse consequences of unprotected sexual activity;
> - ability to access sexual health care;
> - living in an environment that affirms and promotes sexual health.[5]

In the context of men undergoing treatment for prostate cancer (PC), these factors are of critical importance. As changes to sexual health are an expected outcome of treatment, it is essential that men and their partners have an opportunity to be informed of the likelihood of erectile dysfunction, changes to orgasmic function, the potential risk of Peyronie's disease, and the options for rehabilitation. Sexual dysfunction following prostate cancer treatments, particularly after radical prostatectomy (RP), receives greater attention and focus, and may even surpass concerns about cancer recurrence.[6] In comparison to healthy age-matched individuals, prostate cancer patients not only face distressing physical side-effects after RP but also report lower sexual confidence and intimacy levels with their partners. They may experience heightened anxiety related to sexual penetration and perceive a diminished sense of masculinity and self-confidence concerning their sexual abilities following treatment.[7]

In younger men diagnosed with prostate cancer, impacts on fertility are also pertinent with the loss of ejaculate fluid, rendering considerations to long-term fertility management prior to treatment.

5   (World Health Organization, n.d.)
6   (Matthew *et al.*, 2018)
7   (Matthew *et al.*, 2018)

SEXUAL CHANGES AFTER RADICAL PROSTATECTOMY

Sexual changes associated with radical prostatectomy, such as erectile dysfunction, can have a profound impact on both men and their partners. A significant majority of men report experiencing a moderate to severe impact on their overall quality of life as a result.[8]

Parasympathetic neural trauma, along with reduced arterial inflow, increased venous leak, and corporal fibrosis, may contribute to penile hemodynamic changes and penile shortening after RP.[9, 10] These structural changes can persist, leading to additional psychological distress and the potential development of Peyronie's disease. The following are the most frequently reported sexual complaints after RP.

Erectile dysfunction

Erectile dysfunction (ED) is described as the persistent inability to achieve or maintain an erection firm enough or lasting long enough for sexual performance.[11] In 1995, it was estimated to affect 152 million men worldwide with the prevalence expected to double by 2025.[12] Several studies have assessed the epidemiology of ED, with the Massachusetts Aging Study demonstrating increased age as the most significant factor. At age 40 years, approximately 40 percent of men are affected, a rate that increases by 10 percent every decade to age 70. After adjusting for age, it was observed that patients with cardiovascular disease, hypertension, and diabetes had a higher likelihood of experiencing ED during the average assessment period of 8.8 years, as reported by healthcare professionals.[13] Additional recognized risk factors include alcohol use, smoking, depression, pelvic/perineal surgery or trauma, neurological disease, obesity, pelvic radiation, and Peyronie's disease (PD). Hormone deficiency and hypogonadism account for a further 3–5 percent of ED cases, with medications and recreational drugs also affecting erectile function. However, radical prostatectomy has the most significant immediate impact on erectile function, and male patients undergoing the procedure will endure an almost obligatory period of dormancy of the nerves that govern the functional aspect of erection.[14] Although ED is not usually considered a life-threatening condition, it may have significant physical and psychosocial implications that may greatly impact on the quality of life of men and their partners.

The incidence of erectile dysfunction among patients who undergo

---

8   (Chung & Gillman, 2014)
9   (McCullough, 2008)
10 (Montorsi et al., 2004)
11 (Hackett et al., 2018)
12 (Ayta et al., 1999)
13 (Feldman et al., 2000)
14 (Briganti et al., 2004)

radical prostatectomy can vary significantly, similar to urinary incontinence. The available data shows a wide range, with reported rates of ED ranging from 16 percent to 100 percent.[15, 16] The very high proportion of men developing ED following RP is thought to be predominantly caused by nerve damage incurred during surgery.[17] During the RP procedure, the surgeon aims for clear margins and to create a buffer zone between the prostate bed, neurovascular bundle, and rectal tissues, at the same time aiming for total cancer clearance. The proximity of the cavernosal nerve to the prostatic capsule, which is a diffuse and poorly visualized nerve plexus, is adherent to the lateral aspect of the prostate and represents the major surgical obstacle when aiming for minimal nerve damage.[18] The process of removing the prostate inevitably causes cavernosal nerve conductivity problems as well as diminishing the nitric oxide synthesis which is required for mediating smooth muscle relaxation and vasodilation in normal penile erection.[19, 20] Additionally, the likelihood of intracavernosal hypoxia following surgery is considered to be one of the major determinants of post-operative ED. This occurs due to the loss of daily and nocturnal erections with persistent failure of cavernous oxygenation, leading potentially to venous leakage, fibrosis, and penile shortening.[21] Other ED side-effects include the absence of ejaculation due to removal of the ejaculatory duct, orgasmic dysfunction with absent, reduced, or painful orgasms, and climacturia (the loss of urine with any sexual arousal or activity).[22]

Following RP, 60–70 percent of men will have long-term ED, and recovery of function can take up to 48 months.[23] For example, the prostate cancer outcome study revealed that 60 percent of men experienced self-reported ED at 18 months post-RP and about 28 percent of men reported erections with sufficient firmness for penetration at a five-year follow up.[24]

Erectile dysfunction encompasses more than just the inability to achieve penile rigidity sufficient for sexual intercourse. It can also involve various impairments, such as changes in penile function, girth, length, appearance, shape, sensation, strength of erection, and penile pain. In the context of radical prostatectomy, it is reasonable to anticipate an approximate loss of 2–3 cm in penile length within the first 12 months post-surgery.[25]

---

15 (Mulhall *et al.*, 2010)
16 (Dean & Lue, 2005)
17 (Hackett *et al.*, 2018)
18 (Dean & Lue, 2005)
19 (Mulhall *et al.*, 2010)
20 (Dean & Lue, 2005)
21 (Briganti *et al.*, 2004)
22 (Geraerts *et al.*, 2016)
23 (Mulhall, 2009)
24 (Albaugh *et al.*, 2017)
25 (Penson *et al.*, 2008)

Ejaculatory and orgasmic dysfunctions

While substantial research has investigated ED following RP, data available on post-RP orgasmic function is very limited, with almost all available data derived from patients undergoing open surgery and no specific questionnaire for assessment.[26] Complete absence of ejaculate fluid is an immediate side-effect from surgery due to removal of the prostate and seminal vesicles (which account for approximately 90 percent of ejaculate). This may have a profound effect on sexual pleasure at orgasm. In addition, orgasmic changes following RP include absence of orgasm (anorgasmia), alterations in orgasm intensity, orgasmic pain (dysorgasmia), and orgasm-associated urinary incontinence (climacturia). In a small study by Koeman and colleagues only four (29%) from 17 men reported normal orgasmic function following RP, while 50 percent reported a weakened orgasm, 14 percent experienced post-ejaculatory pain and a further 29 percent reported complete loss of orgasm.[27] In a larger cohort of 239 men who underwent open RP, orgasmic function was investigated retrospectively by Barnas and colleagues, and similar findings were made, with 37 percent reporting complete absence of orgasm, 22 percent no change, 37 percent a decrease in orgasm intensity, and dysorgasmia in 14 percent.[28] Of those experiencing pain with ejaculation, 63 percent reported penile pain, 9 percent abdominal pain, and 24 percent rectal pain. A small number of men (4%), however, reported increased orgasm intensity and this has also been recorded by other authors with similar incidence levels.[29] In further studies by Schover and colleagues, 64 percent of men rated themselves distressed about orgasmic function, and this decreased intensity of orgasm (or anorgasmia) has been considered a major psychological distress.[30]

Climacturia

Climacturia, also known as orgasm-associated urinary incontinence, is a prevalent complication that can occur following a radical prostatectomy. However, it is important to note that the reported incidence of climacturia can vary significantly, ranging from 20 percent to 93 percent. [31, 32, 33] In several studies, climacturia rates were higher in patients presenting within 12 months post-RP, with 22 percent reporting leakage at six months and just 9 percent at 24 months.[34] Strategies to help minimize climacturia include encouraging men to empty their bladders prior to sexual activity, use a condom, keep

26 (Salonia et al., 2012)
27 (Koeman et al., 1996)
28 (Barnas et al., 2004)
29 (Barnas et al., 2004)
30 (Schover et al., 2002)
31 (Schover et al., 2002)
32 (Salonia et al., 2012)
33 (Guay & Seftel, 2008)
34 (Lee et al., 2006)

tissues/towels nearby to absorb leakage, and to apply a constriction band at the base of the penis.[35] In cases where climacturia is more challenging to treat, medical intervention involving tricyclic antidepressants and surgical applications of bulbourethral slings have been recommended, and some positive outcomes have been reported.[36] Nevertheless, it is important to highlight that an additional significant approach to managing climacturia is the utilization of pelvic floor muscle (PFM) training techniques, as discussed in Chapter 6. These techniques were initially introduced by Sighinolfi in a case study conducted in 2009,[37] and their effectiveness was further supported by a randomized controlled trial conducted by Geraerts in 2015.[38] In the study, men experiencing climacturia reported improvement or significant reduction after three months of PFM exercises, and these benefits were sustained even at the 12-month post-radical prostatectomy follow-up.[39] The occurrence of orgasm-associated urinary incontinence during various stages of sexual activity, ranging from arousal to post-orgasm, can have a profound impact on individuals and their partners. The effects of this condition can be significant, leading to considerable emotional and psychological distress for those experiencing it.

Psychosexual impairment

Absence of orgasm, decreased orgasm intensity, dysorgasmia, and climacturia may make a man feel uncomfortable, embarrassed, or ashamed.[40] The potential for psychological distress may result in avoidance of sexual activity, loss of self-confidence and self-esteem, and a reduction in quality of life. Changes in sexual desire may decrease by as much as 45 percent in the first six months following RP, causing distress to 60% of participants in Schover's study.[41] Similarly, investigations by Messaoudi stated that 79% of men reported reduced frequency of intercourse post-RP, 76 percent loss of masculine identity, 52 percent loss of self-esteem, and 36 percent anxiety about sexual performance.[42, 43] Given the significant impact of ED causing reduced sexual desire and intimacy, depression and anxiety have been reported in men and their partners post-RP.[44, 45] In a qualitative analysis of 27 PC survivors and their partners by Albaugh, issues of frustration due to changes in sexual

35   (Choi et al., 2007)
36   (Schover et al., 2002)
37   (Sighinolfi et al., 2009)
38   (Geraerts et al., 2016)
39   (Geraerts et al., 2016)
40   (Schover et al., 2002)
41   (Schover et al., 2002)
42   (Messaoudi et al., 2011)
43   (Goldstein et al., 1997)
44   (Nelson et al., 2007)
45   (Chung et al., 2016)

function led to feelings of loss, grief, and in several cases suicidal ideation.[46] Men reported the psychologically devastating effects of feeling abnormal, unnatural, and "less of a man" due to their sexual dysfunction. Both patients and their partners reported that this change had a great impact on every aspect of their lives.

Peyronie's disease

According to ICS Peyronie's disease (PD) is "a connective tissue disorder involving the growth of fibrous plaques in the soft tissue of the penis."[47] It is a symptomatic disorder characterized by a variety of penile symptoms including pain, curvature, shortening, narrowing, indentation, hinge deformity, palpable plaque, and erectile dysfunction. In the general population, PD occurs in 2–9 percent of men, with higher prevalence following prostate cancer treatment.[48, 49] Prostate cancer and Peyronie's disease are commonly observed in men starting from their fifth decade of life. Tal and colleagues conducted a study to establish the incidence of PD among individuals who underwent radical prostatectomy, and identify potential predictors of PD development following the surgical procedure. Their research revealed that approximately 16 percent of the participants were diagnosed with PD.[50]

Following diagnosis and treatment for prostate cancer, the possibility of acquiring PD is not usually discussed in the clinical setting as a potential side-effect. Although sparse, the research that has been undertaken in this area reliably confirms that PD is prevalent following both surgical and radiation approaches in PC. Education for prospective patients should now include this in the general information provided, for the sake of full transparency.

SEXUAL DYSFUNCTION AFTER RADIATION AND ANDROGEN DEPRIVATION THERAPY

While it is acknowledged that prostate cancer survivors who have undergone external beam radiation therapy (EBRT), brachytherapy, and androgen deprivation therapy (ADT) may experience sexual changes, there seems to be a relative lack of emphasis in the existing literature regarding sexual health treatments and overall sexual function for these specific groups. This discrepancy may be attributed to the higher grade of cancers in some patients and a higher incidence of pre-existing comorbidities, which may prevent some interventions.

It is worth noting that although the rates of ED following radical

---

46 (Albaugh, 2010)
47 (Kocjancic *et al.*, 2022)
48 (Chung *et al.*, 2016)
49 (Tal *et al.*, 2010)
50 (Tal *et al.*, 2010)

prostatectomy and radiation therapy are comparable, the onset of ED may often be delayed in patients treated with radiation therapy, as nerve and vessel damage progress.[51] A recent publication, however, shed light on the prevalence and predicting factors for commonly neglected sexual side-effects from EBRT for PC.[52] This included analysis of 109 patients, of whom 12 percent reported an altered curvature in their penis after EBRT. A further 24 percent reported anorgasmia, 44 percent decreased intensity of orgasms, 42 percent penile length loss of >1 cm, 40 percent delayed orgasm, 27 percent decreased sensitivity of the penis, 15 percent orgasm-associated pain, 11 percent pain on ejaculation, 6 percent painful erections, 4 percent climacturia, 2 percent paresthesia, and 2 percent reported a cold sensation. Patients receiving radiation therapies, therefore, are certainly likely to experience far more side-effects than is typically discussed and, once again, education is pivotal to reducing distress.

Most men on ADT treatments may never return to their sexual function baseline levels, as testosterone plays a major role in sexual functioning. Reduced testosterone levels can lead to decreased libido, erectile dysfunction, fewer morning erections, and diminished sexual performance.[53]

SEXUAL FUNCTION ASSESSMENT

It has been proposed that sexual function is best assessed in a naturalistic setting with patient self-report techniques,[54] so most measurements of erectile function are determined by questionnaires. The International Index Erectile Function Score (IIEF-5)[55] and the Expanded Prostate Cancer Index Composite for Clinical Practice (EPIC-CP)[56] are the favored inventories in current scientific publications and cover quality of life, erectile function, and orgasm in men following prostate cancer treatment. The IIEF-5 is a validated measurement tool, and an abridged version of the original 15-point IIEF instrument has been widely used for drug trials. The shorter version is more patient friendly, provides a simple screening measure to supplement medical examination, and is utilized to provide information on symptom severity and impact on the individual. The questionnaire comprises five questions, each ranked 1–5, with a maximum total of 25 indicating normal erectile function. Scores of 1–7 represent severe ED, 8–15 moderate ED, 16–21 mild ED, and 22–25 normal function. For men who have undergone treatment for PC, the EPIC-CP is a more clinically applicable instrument and consists of a one-page,

---

51   (Elliott & Matthew, 2018)
52   (Frey et al., 2017)
53   (Elliott & Matthew, 2018)
54   (Conte, 1983)
55   (Rosen et al., 1997)
56   (Chang et al., 2011)

16-item questionnaire that measures urinary incontinence (UI) and bowel, sexual, and hormonal health-related quality-of-life (HRQoL) domains at the point of care.[57, 58] It has been validated and provides physicians practicing in PC care with improved emphasis and management of patient reported outcomes specifically relating to sexual function, with questions pertaining to quality of erections and orgasm.

TREATMENT OPTIONS
Penile rehabilitation
Penile rehabilitation (PR) is defined as "the use of drug or device to maximize ED recovery" and involves the use of any intervention or combination (medications, devices, or actions) to recover erectile function.[59] The concept of PR was introduced in the 1990s following the introduction of cavernosal nerve-sparing surgeries and the advent of phosphodiesterase type-5 inhibitor (PDE5i) medications, both of which revolutionised approaches to treatment. Subsequently, rehabilitation strategies aim to focus on three interrelated concepts: (1) improving cavernosal oxygenation; (2) preserving endothelial structure and function; (3) preventing smooth muscle structural changes.[60] PR can also have psychological benefits for men during the recovery process, as it can provide them with the ability to achieve an erection through the use of vacuum erection devices or injections. This not only serves a sexual purpose but also offers visual and psychological confirmation that erections are still attainable.[61]

Addressing both erectile dysfunction and the treatment of potential penile deformities is important, and it is now widely recommended to initiate treatment as early as possible after radical prostatectomy to maximize the chances of potential recovery. However, evidence to recommend an irrefutable PR regime has not yet been established, although it is known that over 90 percent of physicians start PR within the first four months post-operatively.[62, 63] The most commonly utilized options for treatment will be outlined below.

Medications: Phosphodiesterase type-5 inhibitors
Medications are used for treatment in PR and include four main PDE5i drugs which are taken orally: Viagra (sildenafil), Levitra (vardenafil), Cialis (tadalafil), and Stendra (avanafil). Since entering the market in 1998, these medications

57 (Chang et al., 2011)
58 (Dean & Lue, 2005)
59 (Mulhall, 2008)
60 (Mulhall, 2008)
61 (Elliott & Matthew, 2018)
62 (Teloken et al., 2009)
63 (Clavell-Hernandez & Wang, 2015)

have been popular amongst physicians and patients, given their safe profile and easy-to-administer approach, with minimal and relatively short lasting side-effects.[64] PDE5i treatments work by decreasing the breakdown of cyclic guanosine monophosphate (cGMP) resulting in elevation of intracellular calcium, causing smooth muscle relaxation and erection, and they have shown favorable outcomes in patients with ED after nerve-sparing RP.[65] In addition, it is acknowledged that the pre-operative status of each individual, including age and erectile function, are well known predictors of post-operative ED and may also alter the impact of functional recovery and, therefore, the impact of PDE5i treatments.[66]

Vacuum erection device

The vacuum erection device (VED) has gained popularity as a treatment option for prostate cancer survivors, regardless of whether they have undergone nerve-sparing radical prostatectomy. It is valued for its low complication rates, minimal side-effects, and cost-effectiveness compared to other options for post-prostatectomy rehabilitation.[67] A recent systematic review has provided evidence of the benefits of using VED in improving sexual function following radical prostatectomy. The study highlighted positive outcomes, including improved International Index of Erectile Function Questionnaire (IIEF-5) scores, preservation of penile length, and satisfactory sexual intercourse when utilizing the vacuum erection device.[68] Early implementation of VED appeared to be effective in preventing penile length loss, enhancing shaft stiffness, and promoting partner satisfaction.[69] Additionally, combining VED with other therapies, such as sildenafil and intracorporeal injections, may further enhance erectile function.[70]

The basic pump design consists of a cylinder which is applied to the flaccid penile shaft and pushed against the patient's pubic region to create an airtight seal.[71] VED activation causes erection by creating a negative pressure around the penis and draws both venous and arterial blood into the corpus cavernosum, resulting in tumescence. ED rings can be used in conjunction with a vacuum pump to prevent the backflow of blood while maintaining an erection and supporting its sustainability. The optimal frequency of VED usage lacks consensus in the literature. However, studies have shown that an early and consistent adherence to a VED program can improve erectile function, particularly following radical prostatectomy. The most commonly

64 (Clavell-Hernandez & Wang, 2015)
65 (Padma-Nathan et al., 2008)
66 (Briganti et al., 2012)
67 (Lin et al., 2015)
68 (Pirola et al., 2023)
69 (Pirola et al., 2023)
70 (Baniel et al., 2001)
71 (Lin et al., 2015)

recommended approach involves daily use of VED for a minimum of six months, either as a standalone therapy or in combination with other treatments.[72] Counseling sessions may play a valuable role in enhancing VED compliance and reducing the likelihood of treatment discontinuation.

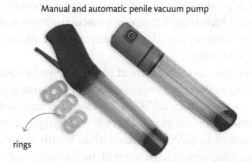

Manual and automatic penile vacuum pump

rings

Intracavernosal injections

Intracavernosal injections (ICI) using alprostadil (prostaglandin E1 derivative), either alone or in combination with papaverine or phentolamine, are a useful treatment for men who have nerve-sparing radical prostatectomy or are unresponsive or cannot tolerate PDE5i medications.[73] When injected directly into the cavernosal tissues, ICIs work primarily on specific receptors found on cavernosal smooth muscle to stimulate the activity of cyclic adenylate cyclase (cAMP) to cause a fall in intracellular calcium and resultant smooth muscle relaxation and erection.[74] Individual doses require gradual adjustment until satisfactory combinations are reached, aiming to have an erection satisfactory for sexual intercourse, but not too long-lasting (>4 hours) to avoid possible priapism.

The first researchers to assess the effectiveness of ICIs in a clinical population were Montorsi and colleagues, who randomized 30 bilateral nerve-sparing post-prostatectomy participants into two groups, to receive either 3 × ICI weekly or none (control) over a 12-week period.[75] At six-month follow-up, 67 percent of men in the treatment group and 20 percent of men in the control group achieved spontaneous erections sufficient for penetration, indicating the likelihood of reduced hypoxia-induced tissue damage with ICI therapy.

Extracorporeal shockwave therapy

Low-intensity extracorporeal shockwave therapy (Li-ESWT) is emerging as a new form of treatment for use in both erectile dysfunction and Peyronie's

---

72 (Pirola *et al.*, 2023)
73 (Montorsi *et al.*, 1997)
74 (Montorsi *et al.*, 1997)
75 (Montorsi *et al.*, 1997)

disease. Its uptake in urology clinics is becoming more widespread and is considered to be a highly favorable treatment option for assisting tissue healing and improved penile function. When Li-ESWT is applied, it carries an energy that can be non-invasively focused to affect a distant selected anatomical region. The shock waves interact with the targeted tissues and induce a cascade of biological reactions, resulting in the release of growth factors and nitric oxide, which trigger tissue neovascularization and a consequent improvement in blood supply, which in turn instigate angiogenesis and new collateral blood channels.

In clinical practice, an earlier form of ESWT known as "radial" shock wave was anticipated to make more improvements than what actually occurred, so a second generation, "focused" ESWT technology has evolved to provide superior outcomes in recent years. There is emerging and strong literature to support the use of Li-ESWT in men with ED, with many clinical studies reporting encouraging results in its use with improved erectile function, good safety records, and short-term durability.[76]

In clinical settings, Li-ESWT treatment for ED is typically provided over 6–10 sessions with direct application to the penis, over a range of sites, and at approximate 20 minutes per session (Figure 10.1). The procedure is painless, but does generate a mild–moderate tingling, "pins and needles" sensation which does not linger beyond the treatment time. Over successive treatments, patients often report an improvement in sensation, penile engorgement, reoccurrence of nocturnal erections, and longer-lasting erections. However, the response to treatment is highly individualized and further research needs to be conducted before there is widespread acceptance of this Li-ESWT technology as the standard of care in ED.

For men seeking improved erectile function following treatment for prostate cancer, research is only in its early days, but anecdotally and small case studies have revealed significant improvements. A recent analysis of the literature in a systematic review that explored nine different clinical trials in this population reported that, despite limited reports due to its new role, low-intensity shockwave therapy after removal of the prostate is a promising non-invasive treatment for dealing with erectile dysfunction after surgery.[77] It was found to be more beneficial in combination with PDE5i medications and at time frames beyond three months after surgery.

Based on the initial findings obtained from preclinical studies conducted on animal models and small clinical trials with short follow-up periods, it can be concluded that Li-ESWT (low-intensity extracorporeal shockwave therapy) may have a potential role in the management of prostate cancer survivors' erectile function. However, it is important to note that larger studies

---

76 (Chung & Wang, 2017)
77 (Sighinolfi *et al.*, 2022)

are necessary to replicate and build upon the existing evidence in this field. These larger studies would provide a more comprehensive understanding of Li-ESWT's efficacy and further validate its potential as a treatment option for post-prostatectomy ED.

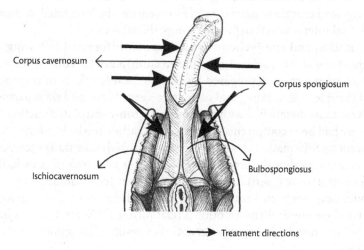

Corpus cavernosum

Corpus spongiosum

Ischiocavernosum

Bulbospongiosus

Treatment directions

FIGURE 10.1: SCHEMATIC OF LI-ESWT APPLICATIONS

Penile prosthetic implants

Penile prosthesis is the most invasive and expensive treatment for ED; however it provides the greatest patient satisfaction (higher than 85%) of all available penile rehabilitation options.[78] Men who underwent implantation reported higher quality of life, erectile function, and frequency of sexual contact, with few side-effects.[79] Several types of prosthesis are available, including a semi-rigid malleable option or an inflatable two- or three-piece device. Sexual functioning is possible within six weeks from surgery, and prevention of long-term penile deformity and penile length are the goals of treatment; however, changes in sensation and ejaculatory function have been reported. In addition, up to 3 percent of patients may acquire infections and penile pain relating to prosthesis sizing errors, erosion, and/or mechanical failure, so long-term management needs to be observed.[80]

Psychosocial therapy

In comparison to biomedical interventions, there is limited research on psychosocial interventions for sexual dysfunction and erectile dysfunction (ED) among prostate cancer survivors. However, studies indicate that sexual

---

78 (Barton *et al.*, 2019)
79 (Goldstein *et al.*, 1997)
80 (Mulcahy, 2010)

counseling and couple-centric psychosocial interventions have the potential to enhance sexual outcomes for both prostate cancer survivors and their partners.[81, 82] Addressing intimacy issues between prostate cancer survivors and their partners is an important aspect of the survivorship experience that cannot be solely addressed through biomedical treatments alone. Therefore, it is suggested that these psychosocial interventions be integrated alongside biomedical interventions to provide comprehensive care.[83]

Education and comprehensive information before and following PC treatment was also considered a significant contributor to reducing distress, and men who were well prepared for the sexual side-effects of treatment found them less devastating and easier to accept.[84] Men and their partners who were most dissatisfied with post-prostatectomy sexual dysfunction felt their care had been compromised by misinformation, too little information, or inaccurate information about the expected sexual dysfunction outcomes.[85] Information regarding the potential for positive sexual experiences, including non-penetrative sex, sensate focus management techniques, and penile rehabilitation, has been found to be highly beneficial for couples aiming to preserve their physical and emotional relationships.[86] Several studies have reported improved relationship strength as a result of incorporating these strategies.[87]

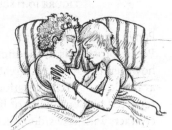

Taking all these aspects into consideration, Salonia and colleagues made a strong recommendation to implement effective psychosexual counseling from the peri-operative stage following PC diagnosis.[88] The authors strongly suggest that patient education should be considered an essential component of the preparations, both prior to and following radical prostatectomy.

A role for therapeutic ultrasound in Peyronie's disease?
Use of therapeutic ultrasound (TUS) in the treatment of soft tissue injuries has origins from the early 1930's, employing high frequency sound waves that utilize mechanical vibration to stimulate tissue repair.[89] It has recently been found to assist in Peyronie's disease in a random controlled trial which

81 (Molton *et al.*, 2008)
82 (Schover *et al.*, 2012)
83 (Matthew *et al.*, 2018)
84 (Albaugh, 2010)
85 (Albaugh, 2010)
86 (Albaugh, 2010)
87 (Chung, 2021)
88 (Salonia *et al.*, 2012)
89 (Speed, 2001)

employed TUS to break down scar tissue, resolve pain, reduce angulation, and improve sexual function in almost 50 participants.[90]

Physiotherapists can easily deliver this treatment, which is non-invasive and delivered over a period of 6–12 sessions for approximately 10 minutess per treatment episode. Protocols include a 1.5–2.5 w/cm^2 intensity to a moderate warmth and a 3MHz frequency.[91] Thermal effects include increased blood flow, reduction in muscle spasm, increased extensibility of collagen fibers, reduction in pain, and a proinflammatory response.[92]

Improvement in the angle of deformity is possibly the most important outcome for patients, given the potential impacts on self-esteem, sexual function, and relationships. There was reported to be an average 17° reduction in curvature; however, several participants who had other penile deformities, such as indentations and hour-glass-shaped formations, also observed improvements in penis shape and appearance.[93]

Additional results from the trial included penile doppler scan measurements pre- and post-TUS sessions to indicate biological change with reductions in penile plaque size. Participants also reported increased capacity for sexual intercourse, reduction in pain for the partner, and overall improved quality of life. [94]

Hence, TUS represents an effective, inexpensive treatment option for men suffering with this difficult-to-treat affliction; it causes no harm, can be provided by any qualified physiotherapist, and may be immediately translated to effective clinical practice.

BIOPSYCHOSOCIAL SEXUAL HEALTH CLINIC MODEL FOR PROSTATE CANCER SURVIVORS AND THEIR PARTNERS, PROPOSED BY MATTHEW ET AL., 2018.[95]
Objectives
The Prostate Cancer Rehabilitation Clinic was developed and made available to men who consented to radical prostatectomy at the Princess Margaret Cancer Centre in Toronto, Ontario, Canada. The objectives were to improve sexual functioning and to support the maintenance of intimacy after RP, addressed by using a biomedical and psychosocial component, through a multidisciplinary biopsychosocial approach.

---

90 (Milios *et al.*, 2020)
91 (Milios *et al.*, 2020)
92 (Speed, 2001)
93 (Milios *et al.*, 2020)
94 (Milios *et al.*, 2020)
95 (Matthew *et al.*, 2018)

Biomedical component

The erectile rehabilitation biomedical component encompassed strategies aimed at facilitating the long-term restoration of erectile function following radical prostatectomy (RP), either with or without the use of erectile agents or devices. The focus was on assisting prostate cancer survivors and their partners in integrating pro-erectile agents into their sexual activity during the recovery process. The treatment plan and prescription were customized to align with the preferences of both patients and couples. An essential aspect of the program was the encouragement for patients and their partners to engage in sexual activity, whether penetrative or non-penetrative, self-stimulation or with a partner, at least once a week. Additionally, initiation of pro-erectile therapy was recommended approximately 6–8 weeks after the RP procedure.

Psychosocial component

The psychosocial component aims to promote intimacy maintenance, utilization of pro-erectile therapy, and regular satisfying sexual activity, whether penetration-based or non-penetration-based. Key topics covered include: education and normalization of sexual health rehabilitation, managing expectations after radical prostatectomy, fostering intimacy and passion, addressing challenges to naturalness and spontaneity, adapting to changes in sexual response, managing performance anxiety, exploring masculinity concerns, addressing grief and loss, addressing partner concerns, enhancing communication and intimacy, understanding the importance of orgasms, incorporating sensate focus techniques, managing sexual desire, adapting to long-term use of pro-erectile therapy, and finding enjoyment in non-penetrative sexual activity. The psychosocial treatment protocol allows for personalization based on the patient's relationship status (single or coupled) and sexual orientation.

Clinic visits

The PCRC program comprised a series of seven clinic visits spanning over a two-year period. These visits include a pre-RP appointment, a consultation with the uro-oncologist approximately 6–8 weeks after the RP procedure, and follow-up appointments with the multi-disciplinary team at 3–4, 7–8, 12–13, 17–18, and 22–24 months post-RP.

"The prostate cancer dance of personal growth": Interview with Brent:
Please state your name, occupation, age, and prostate cancer journey.

Hi, my name is Brent and I am a 62-year-old prostate cancer survivor. I am a counselor therapist who is also involved in spiritual direction, providing space and mental health support for those who have sacred awareness. I was diagnosed with prostate cancer when I was 56, with a Gleason score of 3+3, and was on active surveillance for two years then had a radical prostatectomy in 2020. One year after the surgery, because my PSA kept rising, I had to go on androgen deprivation therapy (ADT) for six months as well as 33 treatments of radiation therapy. My treatments ended in the summer of 2022; since then I have been watching carefully my PSA levels, which seem to be controlled at this time.

Can you describe how you made the decision to have prostatectomy surgery versus other treatment approaches?

Since the beginning of our relationship, I experienced a sense of trust connection with my oncology urologist and surgeon, who elaborated on the specifics for the best practice in prostate cancer treatments. He also suggested that I consult with a radiation oncologist to get their perspective in order to make best informed decisions. Between the two conversations, I felt that it made more sense to opt for the prostatectomy surgery, as it felt safer, cleaner, and could allow for further radiation treatments thereafter if needed. Which in the end was what I needed.

What were the main changes you experienced in your life and your relationship, since your diagnosis and after treatment? What were your main concerns?

"Oh man!" It was quite the shock to be diagnosed with prostate cancer. Especially as I have been healthy all my life and was not experiencing any symptoms whatsoever. It took a while for me to accept that I have this "weakness," and that this relationship with this disease would be a part of my story.

Then I started debating about it: How much research did I want to pursue? How much trust did I have in this particular urologist? Who should I tell? When should I tell my kids? And how much will I freak my family out? It is a pretty big label to share that I have this weakness. I had to decide who I ask for support, who gets included in this process with me, and who gets left out.

After diagnosis, I worried about all possible worse outcomes, for example: losing bladder control, losing muscle mass, and the risks of having potentially no testosterone. Losing sexual function was also a big preoccupation. I expected that as I age there would be a slow decline in sexual function, but this to me felt like my sexual function was dropping off a cliff. I had this quiet nervousness of how my reality will look, as no one can predict.

After treatments there was definitely a sense of weakness, a word "handicap" may come to mind. I used to play a lot of tennis and then I noticed what was a strength before, for example my backhand stroke, was no longer a strength. I used to think to myself: "How is the game going to work now?"

How about your views on your sexuality, masculinity, self-esteem; have they changed since your prostate cancer diagnosis?

Being a white, privileged, cis-gender male, I felt I had a lot of comfort and ease in my life, and after the treatments and diagnosis this ease and confidence in myself was challenged. I had to do a lot of work around my ego and my identity, as I was experiencing this weakness and loss of control.

Going through this cancer journey was a transformative experience for my masculinity, as I had to confront my discomfort in being vulnerable and share my *weakness* around female healthcare professionals and ultimately learn to trust them with my care.

What did you do to overcome some of the distress/ side-effects of prostate cancer diagnosis and treatment? Where did you find support?

I found an article that was quite healing around "dancing with cancer"; it described how cancer is a life dancing partner that you didn't choose, but that you needed to learn how to dance with it and tend to it. This article and finding the meaning to my cancer story helped me find humility to deal with this weakness. I also became a *gentle learner*: learning about the disease, bringing more awareness to my body, and discovering the new roles I can take without a sense of paranoia.

I had never had more support in my life! I am fortunate to live in Canada, and to have access to so many programs and services. Unlike my own experience in Canada with ample post-treatment support, my older brother in the United States—also diagnosed with prostate cancer—had to pay for his radical prostatectomy out-of-pocket and received no support or follow-up care, leaving him to deal with the long-term consequences of the surgery on his own for the past decade.

Very soon after my diagnosis, I found out about a peer navigation program through "True North," where I picked a peer navigator who connected with me through emails and phone calls for about one year.

He shared with me his story without giving me much advice, which I found very healing. I also participated in a few prostate cancer support group meetings, and attended the sexual health and exercise program from the Prostate Cancer Supportive Care (PCSC) Program. I also found support from our visits together, Sam. You helped me gain more understanding about the pelvic floor muscles and some strategies to gain urinary control. Another program that was very valuable to me was the online SHAReClinic, where I was connected with a radiation oncologist who, via conversations, workbooks, and seminars, helped support me for the past two years. I also reached out to counseling professionals to help my mental health status, and invested to have a space to process my emotions and my somatic sensations, as I tend to trick myself by over-functioning and not take care of my emotions.

I am grateful for my wife's unwavering support and love throughout my cancer journey, as she has shown a remarkable balance of being both involved and curious while also providing a gentle and calming presence that allows me to be vulnerable and authentic. My spiritual practices, breath work, and friendships also help me not feel as isolated or alone in this process and have been very life-giving.

Can you describe the role changes that happened in your sexual and emotional relationship with your partner?

This is a very provocative area for me, as I feel dysfunctional and weaker after prostate cancer treatments. After the surgery the penile nerves are touched and go dormant, so I have not been able to have functional erections. However, my wife is healthy and all of a sudden we are not able to play the game that we used to play in our 40 years of marriage. So, there are more vulnerable conversations, maybe focusing more on her pleasure, moving away from the fixed destination of orgasm and being present on the actual whole journey.

We signed up for online classes with Esther Perel to help improve our erotic imagination within our story. This entire situation has actually been refreshing in some ways, forcing us into learning, into a bit of comedy and also a bit of tears. I heard from a seminar I attended that some guys actually quit; if they can't play the field the way they used to play, they just quit, which is very sad. I remember one of the doctors from the SHAReClinic saying that you have to keep showing up and playing, even if you don't feel like it or if it is not working the way you wanted to work. So, I have attempted to continue to play as I believe it is worth trying and learning, even though I am still not in the position of comfort, confidence, and strength yet. I still feel it is important at this stage of our lives to have erotic and intimate touch, so I will continue to pursue it.

Did you pursue any treatments for improving erectile function? Any successes?

Yes I did. I have been working with a sexual health nurse, who has suggested penile rehabilitation using pumps to keep the penile tissue healthy for when the nerves come back. The pump has its use, but unfortunately for me it didn't provide me with sustained erections. The other suggestion was penile injections, and I quote "You have to be kidding me!" After I did some training and learned that it is a very efficacious treatment, with about 90 percent efficacy rate for this particular medication, I decided to give it a go. I have been using this "strange gift" since 2021, allowing me to function and experience pleasure, and at the same time giving pleasure to my wife. Although the penile injection can be an added barrier and is never part of our foreplay, I'm still grateful that it's there.

What kind of transformations and/or growth have you experienced during your prostate cancer journey?

Prostate cancer for me has incentivized me to grow. Dealing with prostate cancer has motivated me to prioritize my health and wellbeing, leading me to adopt a healthier lifestyle without becoming overly obsessive about it: striking a balance and learning to navigate this "cancer dance" without letting it consume my life. I have also found fulfilment in sharing the knowledge and gains I have acquired throughout my prostate cancer journey with others who are navigating this same dance too, recognizing that this journey is not just about my own personal growth, but also about supporting and uplifting others along the way. This cancer path has given me a greater sense of compassion and understanding not only towards my own human condition, but also towards the struggles and challenges faced by others in their own lives.

Do you have any recommendations or suggestions for men, like yourself, going through prostate cancer diagnosis and treatment?

Use all the open doors that come your way and just keep asking for help! That temptation to be self-sufficient and to go "solo" may be very detrimental to this healing process. There are a lot of aids and people to assist and get to know you who can make a significant impact on your life.

I would suggest *not* to do a lot of online research, as it would probably overwhelm you; instead choose to have lots of conversations with health professionals who can direct you to services and programs that are available to you. If you are a prostate cancer patient in Canada, you should take advantage of the numerous resources available to you, which can provide you with invaluable support and guidance throughout your journey at little to no cost.

PROSTATE CANCER SUPPORT PROGRAMS OUTLINED BY BRENT

TrueNTH Peer Navigation Program

The online or phone-based one-on-one support program for Canadians living with prostate cancer is a valuable resource for those seeking personalized guidance and emotional support throughout their cancer journey. The program is administered by experienced prostate cancer survivors who have received extensive training in empathetic listening and are equipped with the knowledge and skills to offer practical advice on managing the disease and its effects. The ultimate goal of the program is to empower patients to become self-reliant and independent in managing their condition, while also providing an additional layer of emotional support that complements the care provided by healthcare professionals.[96]

https://peernavigation.truenth.ca

Prostate Cancer Supportive Care Program

This is a free program for British Columbian (Canada) residents, offering educational and clinical services in primary treatment options, sexual health, exercise, nutrition, androgen deprivation therapy, pelvic floor physiotherapy, counseling services, and metastatic disease management.[97]

https://pcscprogram.ca

TrueNTH SHAReClinic

The Sexual Health and Rehabilitation eClinic is an online biomedical and psychosocial program that connects prostate cancer survivors and their partners with sexual health coaches (e.g., nurses, psychologists, and social workers) to support erectile function and sexual health. The intervention includes online educational modules, online library, and e-visits with sexual health coaches.[98]

https://sharec.truenth.ca

---

96 (True North, n.d.)
97 (Prostate Cancer Supportive Care, n.d.)
98 (Matthew *et al.*, 2022)

Esther Perel's Rekindling Desire

The goal of this pre-recorded video educational class is to facilitate effective communication and improve emotional and sexual satisfaction. Some of the objectives of the course are: understanding personal needs, communicating sexual preferences, understanding barriers, and promoting relational success.

https://rekindlingdesire.estherperel.com

CONCLUSION

Sexual health plays a pivotal role in prostate cancer survivorship due to the significant impact that prostate cancer can have on male sexual wellbeing. Raising awareness and exploring the potential effects of prostate cancer treatments on both physical and psychological aspects of sexual wellbeing may enable men to develop effective coping strategies and embrace their new reality. Emphasizing penile rehabilitation, providing support for intimacy, and involving partners in treatment strategies can enhance sexual health outcomes. By including partners in sexual discussions, physiotherapists and oncology clinicians can adopt a comprehensive and supportive approach to address the challenges faced by patients and their loved ones throughout the treatment journey. Early education about opportunities for positive sexual experiences and information on potential sexual side-effects of treatment can be instrumental in strengthening the physical and emotional bond between prostate cancer survivors and their partners, ultimately enhancing their overall cancer experience.

REFERENCES

Albaugh, J.A. (2010). Addressing and managing erectile dysfunction after prostatectomy for prostate cancer. *Urologic Nursing, 30*(3), 167–177, 166. https://doi.org/10.7257/1053-816X.2010.30.3.167

Albaugh, J.A., Sufrin, N., Lapin, B.R., Petkewicz, J., & Tenfelde, S. (2017). Life after prostate cancer treatment: A mixed methods study of the experiences of men with sexual dysfunction and their partners. *BMC Urology, 17*(1), 45. https://doi.org/10.1186/s12894-017-0231-5

Ayta, I.A., McKinlay, J.B., & Krane, R.J. (1999). The likely worldwide increase in erectile dysfunction between 1995 and 2025 and some possible policy consequences. *BJU International, 84*(1), 50–56. https://doi.org/10.1046/j.1464-410x.1999.00142.x

Baniel, J., Israilov, S., Segenreich, E., & Livne, P.M. (2001). Comparative evaluation of treatments for erectile dysfunction in patients with prostate cancer after radical retropubic prostatectomy. *BJU International, 88*(1), 58–62. https://doi.org/10.1046/j.1464-410x.2001.02254.x

Barnas, J.L., Pierpaoli, S., Ladd, P., Valenzuela, R., et al. (2004). The prevalence and nature of orgasmic dysfunction after radical prostatectomy. *BJU International, 94*(4), 603–605. https://doi.org/10.1111/j.1464-410X.2004.05009.x

Barton, G.J., Carlos, E.C., & Lentz, A.C. (2019). Sexual quality of life and satisfaction with penile prostheses. *Sexual Medicine Reviews*, 7(1), 178–188. https://doi.org/10.1016/j.sxmr.2018.10.003

Briganti, A., Salonia, A., Zanni, G., Fabbri, F., *et al.* (2004). Erectile dysfunction and radical prostatectomy: An update. *EAU Update Series*, 2(2), 84–92. https://doi.org/10.1016/j.euus.2004.03.003

Briganti, A., Di Trapani, E., Abdollah, F., Gallina, A., *et al.* (2012). Choosing the best candidates for penile rehabilitation after bilateral nerve-sparing radical prostatectomy. *Journal of Sexual Medicine*, 9(2), 608–617. https://doi.org/10.1111/j.1743-6109.2011.02580.x

Chang, P., Szymanski, K.M., Dunn, R.L., Chipman, J.J., *et al.* (2011). Expanded prostate cancer index composite for clinical practice: Development and validation of a practical, health related, quality of life instrument for use in the routine clinical care of patients with prostate cancer. *Journal of Urology*, 186(3), 865–872. https://doi.org/10.1016/j.juro.2011.04.085

Choi, J.M., Nelson, C.J., Stasi, J., & Mulhall, J.P. (2007). Orgasm associated incontinence (climacturia) following radical pelvic surgery: Rates of occurrence and predictors. *Journal of Urology*, 177(6), 2223–2226. https://doi.org/10.1016/j.juro.2007.01.150

Chung, E. (2021). Male sexual dysfunction and rehabilitation strategies in the settings of salvage prostate cancer treatment. *International Journal of Impotence Research*, 33(4), Article 4. https://doi.org/10.1038/s41443-021-00437-4

Chung, E., & Gillman, M. (2014). Prostate cancer survivorship: A review of erectile dysfunction and penile rehabilitation after prostate cancer therapy. *Medical Journal of Australia*, 200(10), 582–585. https://doi.org/10.5694/mja13.11028

Chung, E., & Wang, J. (2017). A state-of-art review of low intensity extracorporeal shock wave therapy and lithotripter machines for the treatment of erectile dysfunction. *Expert Review of Medical Devices*, 14(12), 929–934. https://doi.org/10.1080/17434440.2017.1403897

Chung, E., Ralph, D., Kagioglu, A., Garaffa, G., *et al.* (2016). Evidence-based management guidelines on Peyronie's Disease. *Journal of Sexual Medicine*, 13(6), 905–923. https://doi.org/10.1016/j.jsxm.2016.04.062

Clavell-Hernandez, J., & Wang, R. (2015). Penile rehabilitation following prostate cancer treatment: Review of current literature. *Asian Journal of Andrology*, 17(6), 916–922; discussion 921. https://doi.org/10.4103/1008-682X.150838

Conte, H.R. (1983). Development and use of self-report techniques for assessing sexual functioning: A review and critique. *Archives of Sexual Behavior*, 12(6), 555–576. https://doi.org/10.1007/BF01542217

Danoff, D.S. (2011). *Penis Power: The Ultimate Guide to Male Sexual Health, 1st edition.* New York: Del Monaco Press.

Dean, R.C., & Lue, T.F. (2005). Physiology of penile erection and pathophysiology of erectile dysfunction. *Urologic Clinics of North America*, 32(4), 379–395, v. https://doi.org/10.1016/j.ucl.2005.08.007

Elliott, S., & Matthew, A. (2018). Sexual recovery following prostate cancer: Recommendations from two established Canadian sexual rehabilitation clinics. *Sexual Medicine Reviews*, 6(2), 279–294. https://doi.org/10.1016/j.sxmr.2017.09.001

Feldman, H.A., Johannes, C.B., Derby, C.A., Kleinman, K.P., Mohr, B.A., Araujo, A.B., & McKinlay, J.B. (2000). Erectile dysfunction and coronary risk factors: Prospective results from the Massachusetts male aging study. *Preventive Medicine*, 30(4), 328–338. https://doi.org/10.1006/pmed.2000.0643

Frey, A., Pedersen, C., Lindberg, H., Bisbjerg, R., Sønksen, J., & Fode, M. (2017). Prevalence and predicting factors for commonly neglected sexual side-effects to external-beam radiation therapy for prostate cancer. *Journal of Sexual Medicine*, 14(4), 558–565. https://doi.org/10.1016/j.jsxm.2017.01.015

Geraerts, I., Van Poppel, H., Devoogdt, N., De Groef, A., Fieuws, S., & Van Kampen, M. (2016). Pelvic floor muscle training for erectile dysfunction and climacturia one year after nerve-sparing radical prostatectomy: A randomized controlled trial. *International Journal of Impotence Research*, 28(1), Article 1. https://doi.org/10.1038/ijir.2015.24

Goldstein, I., Newman, L., Baum, N., Brooks, M., *et al.* (1997). Safety and efficacy outcome of mentor alpha-1 inflatable penile prosthesis implantation for impotence treatment. *Journal of Urology*, *157*(3), 833–839. https://doi.org/10.1097/00005392-199703000-00023

Guay, A., & Seftel, A.D. (2008). Sexual foreplay incontinence in men with erectile dysfunction after radical prostatectomy: A clinical observation. *International Journal of Impotence Research*, *20*(2), 199–201. https://doi.org/10.1038/sj.ijir.3901609

Hackett, G., Kirby, M., Wylie, K., Heald, A., Ossei-Gerning, N., Edwards, D., & Muneer, A. (2018). British Society for Sexual Medicine guidelines on the management of erectile dysfunction in men-2017. *Journal of Sexual Medicine*, *15*(4), 430–457. https://doi.org/10.1016/j.jsxm.2018.01.023

Kocjancic, E., Chung, E., Garzon, J.A., Haylen, B., *et al.* (2022). International Continence Society (ICS) report on the terminology for sexual health in men with lower urinary tract (LUT) and pelvic floor (PF) dysfunction. *Neurourology and Urodynamics*, *41*(1), 140–165. https://doi.org/10.1002/nau.24846

Koeman, M., van Driel, M.F., Schultz, W.C., & Mensink, H.J. (1996). Orgasm after radical prostatectomy. *British Journal of Urology*, *77*(6), 861–864. https://doi.org/10.1046/j.1464-410x.1996.01416.x

Lee, J., Hersey, K., Lee, C.T., & Fleshner, N. (2006). Climacturia following radical prostatectomy: Prevalence and risk factors. *The Journal of Urology*, *176*(6), 2562–2565. https://doi.org/10.1016/j.juro.2006.07.158

Lin, H., Wang, G., & Wang, R. (2015). [Application of the vacuum erectile device in penile rehabilitation for erectile dysfunction after radical prostatectomy]. *Zhonghua Nan Ke Xue* [*National Journal of Andrology*], *21*(3), 195–199. http://dx.doi.org/10.3978/j.issn.2223-4683.2013.01.04

Matthew, A., Lutzky-Cohen, N., Jamnicky, L., Currie, K., *et al.* (2018). The Prostate Cancer Rehabilitation Clinic: A biopsychosocial clinic for sexual dysfunction after radical prostatectomy. *Current Oncology*, *25*(6), 393–402. https://doi.org/10.3747/co.25.4111

Matthew, A.G., Trachtenberg, L.J., Yang, Z.G., Robinson, J., *et al.* (2022). An online Sexual Health and Rehabilitation eClinic (TrueNTH SHAReClinic) for prostate cancer patients: A feasibility study. *Supportive Care in Cancer*, *30*(2), 1253–1260. https://doi.org/10.1007/s00520-021-06510-4

McCullough, A. (2008). Penile change following radical prostatectomy: Size, smooth muscle atrophy, and curve. *Current Urology Reports*, *9*(6), 492–499. https://doi.org/10.1007/s11934-008-0084-2

Messaoudi, R., Menard, J., Ripert, T., Parquet, H., & Staerman, F. (2011). Erectile dysfunction and sexual health after radical prostatectomy: Impact of sexual motivation. *International Journal of Impotence Research*, *23*(2), 81–86. https://doi.org/10.1038/ijir.2011.8

Milios, J.E., Ackland, T.R., & Green, D.J. (2020). Peyronie's disease and the role of therapeutic ultrasound: A randomized controlled trial. *Journal of Rehabilitation Therapy*, *2*(2). www.rehabiljournal.com/articles/peyronies-disease-and-the-role-of-therapeutic-ultrasound-a-randomized-controlled-trial.html

Molton, I.R., Siegel, S.D., Penedo, F.J., Dahn, J.R., *et al.* (2008). Promoting recovery of sexual functioning after radical prostatectomy with group-based stress management: The role of interpersonal sensitivity. *Journal of Psychosomatic Research*, *64*(5), 527–536. https://doi.org/10.1016/j.jpsychores.2008.01.004

Montorsi, F., Guazzoni, G., Strambi, L.F., Da Pozzo, L.F., *et al.* (1997). Recovery of spontaneous erectile function after nerve-sparing radical retropubic prostatectomy with and without early intracavernous injections of alprostadil: Results of a prospective, randomized trial. *Journal of Urology*, *158*(4), 1408–1410. http://dx.doi.org/10.1016/S0022-5347(01)64227-7

Montorsi, F., Briganti, A., Salonia, A., Rigatti, P., & Burnett, A.L. (2004). Current and future strategies for preventing and managing erectile dysfunction following radical prostatectomy. *European Urology*, *45*(2), 123–133. https://doi.org/10.1016/j.eururo.2003.08.016

Mulcahy, J.J. (2010). Current approach to the treatment of penile implant infections. *Therapeutic Advances in Urology*, *2*(2), 69–75. https://doi.org/10.1177/1756287210370330

Mulhall, J.P. (2008). Penile rehabilitation following radical prostatectomy. *Current Opinion in Urology*, *18*(6), 613. https://doi.org/10.1097/MOU.0b013e3283136462

Mulhall, J.P. (2009). Defining and reporting erectile function outcomes after radical prostatectomy: Challenges and misconceptions. *Journal of Urology, 181*(2), 462–471. https://doi.org/10.1016/j.juro.2008.10.047

Mulhall, J.P., Parker, M., Waters, B.W., & Flanigan, R. (2010). The timing of penile rehabilitation after bilateral nerve-sparing radical prostatectomy affects the recovery of erectile function. *BJU International, 105*(1), 37–41. https://doi.org/10.1111/j.1464-410X.2009.08775.x

National Cancer Institute (NCI) (2011). Definition of sexuality. Retrieved September 22, 2023, from www.cancer.gov/publications/dictionaries/cancer-terms/def/sexuality

Nelson, C.J., Choi, J.M., Mulhall, J.P., & Roth, A.J. (2007). Determinants of sexual satisfaction in men with prostate cancer. *Journal of Sexual Medicine, 4*(5), 1422–1427. https://doi.org/10.1111/j.1743-6109.2007.00547.x

Oswald, F., Khera, D., & Pedersen, C.L. (2021). The association of genital appearance satisfaction, penis size importance, and penis-centric masculinity to chronically discriminatory ideologies among heterosexual men. *Psychology of Men & Masculinities, 22*(4), 704–714. https://doi.org/10.1037/men0000360

Padma-Nathan, H., McCullough, A.R., Levine, L.A., Lipshultz, L.I., *et al.* (2008). Randomized, double-blind, placebo-controlled study of postoperative nightly sildenafil citrate for the prevention of erectile dysfunction after bilateral nerve-sparing radical prostatectomy. *International Journal of Impotence Research, 20*(5), 479–486. https://doi.org/10.1038/ijir.2008.33

Penson, D.F., McLerran, D., Feng, Z., Li, L., *et al.* (2008). Five-year urinary and sexual outcomes after radical prostatectomy: Results from the Prostate Cancer Outcomes Study. *Journal of Urology, 179*(5 Suppl), S40–S44. https://doi.org/10.1016/j.juro.2008.03.136

Pirola, G.M., Naselli, A., Maggi, M., Gubbiotti, M., *et al.* (2023). Vacuum erection device for erectile function rehabilitation after radical prostatectomy: Which is the correct schedule? Results from a systematic, scoping review. *International Journal of Impotence Research.* https://doi.org/10.1038/s41443-023-00700-w

Prostate Cancer Supportive Care (n.d.). About. Retrieved April 3, 2023, from https://pcscprogram.ca/pcsc-program/about

Rosen, R.C., Riley, A., Wagner, G., Osterloh, I.H., Kirkpatrick, J., & Mishra, A. (1997). The international index of erectile function (IIEF): A multidimensional scale for assessment of erectile dysfunction. *Urology, 49*(6), 822–830. https://doi.org/10.1016/s0090-4295(97)00238-0

Salonia, A., Burnett, A.L., Graefen, M., Hatzimouratidis, K., Montorsi, F., Mulhall, J.P., & Stief, C. (2012). Prevention and management of postprostatectomy sexual dysfunctions part 2: Recovery and preservation of erectile function, sexual desire, and orgasmic function. *European Urology, 62*(2), 273–286. https://doi.org/10.1016/j.eururo.2012.04.047

Schover, L.R., Fouladi, R.T., Warneke, C.L., Neese, L., Klein, E.A., Zippe, C., & Kupelian, P.A. (2002). Defining sexual outcomes after treatment for localized prostate carcinoma. *Cancer, 95*(8), 1773–1785. https://doi.org/10.1002/cncr.10848

Schover, L.R., Canada, A.L., Yuan, Y., Sui, D., Neese, L., Jenkins, R., & Rhodes, M.M. (2012). A randomized trial of internet-based versus traditional sexual counseling for couples after localized prostate cancer treatment. *Cancer [ISSN:0008543X], 118*(2), 500–509. https://doi.org/10.1002/cncr.26308

Sighinolfi, M.C., Rivalta, M., Mofferdin, A., Micali, S., De Stefani, S., & Bianchi, G. (2009). Potential effectiveness of pelvic floor rehabilitation treatment for postradical prostatectomy incontinence, climacturia, and erectile dysfunction: A case series. *Journal of Sexual Medicine, 6*(12). https://doi.org/10.1111/j.1743-6109.2009.01493.x

Sighinolfi, M.C., Eissa, A., Bellorofonte, C., Mofferdin, A., *et al.* (2022). Low-intensity Extracorporeal Shockwave Therapy for the management of postprostatectomy erectile dysfunction: A systematic review of the literature. *European Urology Open Science, 43*, 45–53. https://doi.org/10.1016/j.euros.2022.07.003

Speed, C.A. (2001). Therapeutic ultrasound in soft tissue lesions. *Rheumatology (Oxford, England), 40*(12), 1331–1336. https://doi.org/10.1093/rheumatology/40.12.1331

Tal, R., Heck, M., Teloken, P., Siegrist, T., Nelson, C.J., & Mulhall, J.P. (2010). Peyronie's disease following radical prostatectomy: Incidence and predictors. *Journal of Sexual Medicine, 7*(3), 1254–1261. https://doi.org/10.1111/j.1743-6109.2009.01655.x

Teloken, P., Mesquita, G., Montorsi, F., & Mulhall, J. (2009). Post-radical prostatectomy pharmacological penile rehabilitation: Practice patterns among the International Society for Sexual Medicine Practitioners. *Journal of Sexual Medicine, 6*(7), 2032–2038. https://doi.org/10.1111/j.1743-6109.2009.01269.x

Tolman, D.L., & Diamond, L.M. (2001). Desegregating sexuality research: Cultural and biological perspectives on gender and desire. *Annual Review of Sex Research, 12*(1), 33–74. https://doi.org/10.1080/10532528.2001.10559793

True North (n.d.). Welcome to peer navigation. Retrieved April 21, 2023, from https://peer-navigation.truenth.ca

World Health Organization (WHO) (n.d.). Sexual health. Retrieved May 23, 2023, from www.who.int/health-topics/sexual-health

CHAPTER 11

The Social Part 2: Social Support

Humans are social beings and are defined by social interactions and a sense of belonging. As per the *belongingness hypothesis,* human beings from all cultures have an innate need to form and maintain positive bonds and relationships, influencing their cognition, emotions, and behavior.[1] According to the World Happiness Report, happiness is more related to the quality of people's interactions than with income, 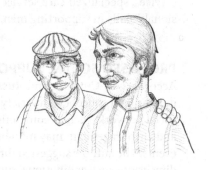 once basic economic needs are met.[2] Meik Wiking, the author of *The Little Book of Hygge* and the CEO of the Happiness Institute in Denmark, reported that the more satisfied people are with their human connections, the more satisfied they are with their lives.[3] It was noted that Danish people's experience of *togetherness,* which is embedded in their social rituals, may promote creativity, democracy, inclusion, and a sense of belonging, contributing to high levels of reported happiness.[4]

There are numerous studies linking social support and social integration as a landmark for health.[5] Social isolation and seclusion can particularly affect older adults' wellbeing and mental and physical health. For example, older adults who live alone and express feelings of loneliness may have greater risks of cognitive decline, decreased ability to perform activities of daily living, and increased health problems.[6] In addition, older adults with strong family and friend networks may be more likely to engage in recreational activities, further improving their sense of wellbeing and healthy living.[7]

Increased social support in cancer care has been linked to improved

---

1   (Baumeister & Leary, 1995)
2   (World Happiness Report, n.d.)
3   (Wiking, 2016)
4   (Lee *et al.*, 2020)
5   (Costanzo *et al.*, 2011)
6   (Fernandez-Portero *et al.*, 2023)
7   (Fernandez-Portero *et al.*, 2023)

mental status and better quality of life, and shown to improve morbidity and mortality.[8, 9, 10] Additionally, social support can be an effective way of coping with stress attributed to cancer. According to the *transaction model of stress and coping*, which suggests that stress coping strategies arise from the interplay between individuals and their environment,[11] seeking social support may facilitate emotion- or problem-focused strategies to improve cancer-related stress.[12]

Socially supporting prostate cancer survivors may include peer support access, community involvement and advocacy, family and partner supportive services, specialized care service availability, and improving health professionals' skills in supporting men.[13]

PROPOSED SOCIAL SUPPORT CLASSIFICATION

According to Cutrona and Russel,[14] social support seems to be a multi-dimensional concept, as a variety of interpersonal interactions from people's social network, such as companionship, direct care, expression of affection, and encouragement, may influence their coping strategies after adverse life events. The authors suggested further classifying social support into different dimensions such as emotional support, social integration or network support, esteem support, tangible aid, informational support, and opportunity for nurturance:

- *Emotional support* is the support received from others for comfort and security, and resulting in the feeling of being cared for.
- *Social integration* results in the feeling of commonality, of being part of a group with shared interests or concerns, which may result in increased recreational activities and participation.
- *Esteem support* is the support received to enable someone's self-esteem and confidence; for example, receiving positive feedback for one's abilities or expressing belief in one's successful coping strategies.
- *Tangible aid* is receiving concrete instrumental assistance such as monetary assistance or physical help.
- *Informational support* is receiving guidance for addressing a concern or a difficulty.
- *Opportunity to provide nurturance* is the action of giving support to

---

8 (Zhao *et al.*, 2021)
9 (Colloca & Colloca, 2016)
10 (Costanzo *et al.*, 2011)
11 (Mukwato *et al.*, 2010)
12 (Lazarus & Folkman, 1984)
13 (Dunn *et al.*, 2020)
14 (Cutrona & Russell, 1990)

others, which may enhance the supporter's feelings of being needed by others, or the experience of a sense of personal competence.

PROSTATE CANCER AND SOCIAL SUPPORT

Prostate cancer is a disease that may affect patients and their families emotionally, financially, and behaviorally. Prostate cancer diagnosis, treatments, and side-effects can particularly affect younger patients' family functioning by challenging parental roles, family dynamics, and sexual relationships.[15] The impact of diagnosis and undergoing radical treatments (prostatectomy and radiotherapy) may also result in relationship strains between the patients and their partners, due to uncertainty and anxiety after diagnosis and functional changes post-treatment.[16]

Considering that quality-of-life satisfaction may predict prostate cancer's overall survival rate,[17] psychosocial interventions in clinical settings should be prioritized. Social support, defined by many as the degree of perceived satisfaction with their social relationships, has many psychological benefits in cancer care. It may foster resilience and optimism, which have been shown to improve self-efficacy, and health-related quality of life in prostate cancer survivors upon diagnosis.[18] Physiologically, social support interventions were shown to have an effect on upregulating immune cell responses (particularly NK-cells) and down-regulating cell stress responses, which may have an effect on inhibiting tumor progression and metastasis.[19]

Added familial support and integrating family members in psychosocial interventions seems to have a positive effect on psychological distress of cancer patients.[20] Prostate cancer survivors with many friends or family members to share emotional problems with may have decreased stress levels compared to those with few or no friends or family members.[21] In Chinese society, where the importance of family relationships is very high and forms the foundation of their social organizations, increased perceived family support was strongly correlated with decreased prostate cancer patients' depressive symptoms.[22] Additionally, partner support at prostate cancer diagnosis seems to have positive effects on both partners' relationship satisfaction and mental quality of life, between diagnosis and six months.[23] In metastatic prostate cancer patients, social and familiar wellbeing, including caregiver's clinic

15   (Collaço et al., 2019)
16   (Vyas et al., 2022)
17   (Colloca & Colloca, 2016)
18   (Cuypers et al., 2018)
19   (Costanzo et al., 2011)
20   (Martire et al., 2004)
21   (Jan et al., 2016)
22   (Zhao et al., 2021)
23   (Varner et al., 2019)

visit involvement, was associated with psychological wellness, information competency, need fulfilment, and overall satisfaction.[24]

In prostatectomy patients, added social support to a pelvic floor muscle exercise program was shown to improve home program engagement, urinary outcomes, and quality-of-life domains such as spousal relationship and social outings.[25] Group programs that facilitate social support may contribute to enhanced exercise programs' physiological and psychological effects, including exercise adherence.

PEER SUPPORT

Peer support is a non-hierarchical empathic type of support given and received by individuals who share similar experiences, health concerns, or challenges. It is a "system of giving and receiving help founded on key principles of respect, shared responsibility, and mutual agreement of what is helpful."[26] Peer support may be given via one-on-one conversations, formal or informal group meetings, or online communities and networks.

Peer support programs can complement or provide an alternative support option to healthcare services, may aid in suicide prevention,[27] promote the wellbeing of people receiving or delivering it, and improve participants' self-esteem, sense of control, and acceptance.[28] Peer support in cancer care may help decrease negative effects of the disease on general health, coping capacities, relationships, and functions of daily living.[29] In prostate cancer care, engaging in peer support programs may address and enhance emotional support, social integration, esteem support, and informational support, and create opportunities for nurturance.

Since the 1990s, prostate cancer peer support groups (PCSGs) from all over the world have formed to facilitate men's coping with the illness and its side-effects. These support groups are usually associated with or advertised by cancer patient foundations, organizations, or associations. Prostate cancer peer support workers, who usually are volunteers placing themselves as group leaders and advocates for the disease, facilitate these activities and meetings with duties such as listening, providing hope, sharing experiences and thoughts, and providing informed knowledge on healthcare systems, cancer, and men's health.[30] Information seeking seems to be the most common reason why prostate cancer patients and family members attend prostate cancer

---

24 (Colloca & Colloca, 2016)
25 (Zhang et al., 2007)
26 (Mead et al., 2001)
27 (Schlichthorst et al., 2020)
28 (Jones & Pietilä, 2020)
29 (Jones & Pietilä, 2020)
30 (Jones & Pietilä, 2020)

support groups.[31] Denial of illness, privacy concerns, perception of weakness or fear of stigmatization, ignorance of what PCSGs may offer, and difficulty with access may be some of the barriers for men not to attend prostate cancer support groups.[32] Language barriers and different cultural values may also influence men who do not attend a PCSG.[33]

GROUP EXERCISE PROGRAMS

Fitness groups or exercise programs geared towards prostate cancer survivors may facilitate physiological benefits and social support. Although there aren't many studies evaluating the effectiveness of group programs in improving social support of prostate cancer survivors, these group programs may be a contributing environment for sharing information, developing emotional connections, and improving physical and mental health. It may be more beneficial for some to participate in "action-oriented" group programs that may give prostate cancer survivors the same opportunities to exchange information and share experiences as talk-based support group programs.[34]

A pilot randomized control study (my study, unpublished, 2014) of a group physiotherapy program post-prostatectomy demonstrated good acceptability, high attendance rates, increased social support, and improved burden of urinary incontinence. Some of the main themes extracted in this study after completion of the group program were "increased social support" and "helpful to share and listen to others' experiences and stories." This study also demonstrated that post-prostatectomy, men with urinary incontinence when exposed to a positive and open environment can be motivated to attend a physiotherapist-led group program and to be open to discuss intimate issues with the physiotherapist and each other.

Palliative cancer patients attending a supervised group exercise program reported increased social connection, perception of health, sense of belonging, and coping.[35] This qualitative study reported on how palliative cancer patients, when exercising with other palliative cancer patients, expressed an improved sense of belonging by being able to connect with people that "are in the same boat."[36]

---

31 (Garrett *et al.*, 2014)
32 (Garrett *et al.*, 2014)
33 (Garrett *et al.*, 2014)
34 (Paltiel *et al.*, 2009)
35 (Paltiel *et al.*, 2009)
36 (Paltiel *et al.*, 2009)

"Exercising with prostate cancer buddies": Interview with Neil:
Please tell me your name, age, occupation, and prostate cancer survivorship path.

My name is Neil and I am a 64-year-old sailor and retired mechanical engineering technologist. I was an aircraft maintainer in the Royal Canadian Air Force and an instructor in the mechanical engineering department at Camosun College (British Columbia). I was diagnosed with inoperable high-risk prostate cancer (Gleason score of 4+5) on January 3, 2017 at 5 pm (I remember this date very well). Since then, I have been going through a plethora of therapies, including hormonal treatments (bicalutamide, leuprorelin, goserelin, and apalutamide), external beam radiation therapy, high dose brachytherapy, and recently stereotactic ablative radiotherapy (SABR) as the hormonal drugs weren't working anymore. SABR was "brutal": I had a lot of bowel issues, and only just recently—in the past month—I am starting to feel myself again.

Currently, I am considered a palliative prostate cancer patient, and have been told that I may have one to two years of living. As difficult as it is to hear this news, I am trying to make the most of the time I have left, and am determined to beat the odds.

What are the main side-effects you have experienced since your treatments? Are the side-effects affecting your motivation to move or exercise?

Following the start of my hormonal therapy, I experienced weight gain and also noticed difficulty concentrating and fogginess during the first course of treatment, which left me uncertain whether the mental changes were due to the medication's side-effects or if they indicated a decline in my mental health. To address these concerns, I consulted with a psychiatrist who prescribed me an antidepressant medication that proved immensely helpful. My mental change after I started taking the antidepressant was akin to being out at sea on a foggy day, when suddenly the fog dissipates and everything is suddenly clear and visible.

Currently, I find myself contending with various aches and pains—which I'm uncertain whether they are related to my cancer or simply a byproduct of ageing— as well as *persistent fatigue*. I used to be a very fit individual before diagnosis, as I rode my bike to work, played squash, and exercised all my life. My father was an exercise "sergeant," so exercising was embedded in my upbringing. But now I feel very tired, especially when I exert myself, and find myself needing to rest more frequently. As an example: yesterday, I went sailing and encountered challenging conditions as the wind unexpectedly intensified to over 20 knots, making it difficult for my body to keep pace with the boat, ultimately leading us to call it quits. After the sailing I was definitely very tired.

Despite experiencing fatigue, I remain committed to my weekly routine, which includes walking for about 4–5 kilometers, engaging in woodworking, helping my wife with gardening, and sailing.

When did you join the exercise group program, how did you find out about it, and what motivated you to attend?

In 2017, the exercise class was recommended to me by the Island Prostate Centre following my brachytherapy, and that's when I decided to join the exercise class. Joining a fitness class for me was important because, first of all, I wanted to be motivated to lose weight (as after I started hormone therapy I have gained 30 pounds), and second of all, for me being physically fit meant being able to carry on with life the best way possible. Being a highly social individual, I was also driven to seek out a community of like-minded individuals who may be encountering similar life events to mine.

When I went back for treatment in November 2022, I stopped attending the fitness class.

Can you describe to me the type of exercises you did, how big the classes were, how many times a week, for how long, and how were the participants' fitness levels? Where did the classes take place, and what was the environment like?

The classes were offered in-person twice a week for about one hour, each class in a community college fitness area and in a rental hall. We usually had a warm-up session and then it would break up into a strength training circuit class (do it yourself kind of style), ending with stretching and meditative breathing sessions. The instructors were always there to guide us through various techniques and provide the necessary encouragement, especially since there was often a lot of chatting going on. Every session consisted of a group of 8 to 15 men, ranging from their mid-50s to late-70s, who varied in their fitness levels and abilities. The class was marked by a great sense of camaraderie, as the like-minded individuals present were always eager to lend their support and encouragement, making for a positive and light-hearted atmosphere.

Since the pandemic in 2020, the classes went to Zoom and many participants dropped out, as it wasn't the same environment as the in-person classes, especially as some of them were more engaged to attend due to the social aspect of the class. The Zoom classes probably have enhanced the physical nature of the fitness classes because there was less time for socializing and chit-chatting.

What was the experience like for you while attending the group classes? What were the benefits you noticed while and after attending the classes? What kept you motivated to attend?

During the time that I attended the group classes, I was undergoing a significant emotional struggle, but the group classes provided me with a much-needed source of positive energy. Upon finishing each session, I distinctly recall feeling a sense of upliftment and positive energy that stayed with me long after leaving the class. The classes offered a *profound sense of support*, which was particularly crucial given the daunting and frightening nature of a cancer diagnosis—for instance, when someone, who may receive a diagnosis of having only six months to live without treatment, could attend class and discover that several individuals present had also received similar news, yet had been fighting cancer successfully for five to six years.

I also developed personal relationships with some of the instructors and made lifelong friendships with some of the participants in the group class. Because of the structure of the class, seeing the same people week to week allowed us to begin new routines, for example, going for lunch after the class, and even meeting up outside of the classes for social engagements.

In my opinion, the fitness group classes served as a kind of hook or pretext for men to gather together and discuss their cancer experiences, as they might not have otherwise found an opportunity or felt comfortable enough to broach the topic. In my case, the in-person fitness group class truly made a difference in my life.

How does the support received from attending a fitness group class differ, if at all, from the support provided in a support group meeting?

In my opinion the prostate cancer support meeting and the group exercise program are both valuable. However, one is very different from the other. In the support group meetings, I had the opportunity to gain *informational support* from a diverse range of healthcare experts, who provided valuable guidance on various aspects related to cancer management, such as nutrition recommendations, and the latest developments in prostate cancer treatment options. The in-person exercise group programs offer informational support as well as a unique opportunity to foster a sense of community and social connection, as the regular bi-weekly meetings and consistent participation of both staff and attendees creates a supportive and safe environment that encourages conversation and sharing.

How are you feeling now and what are your plans for the future?

Regardless of experiencing occasional bouts of fatigue that leave me feeling drained and unable to engage in much physical activity, I'm beginning to feel like I'm recovering from my previous treatments, and I'm eager to rejoin the exercise classes. The current mode of delivery for the fitness classes is still via Zoom, which in my opinion is far from ideal. I think the main challenge being faced right now in returning to an in-person group setting is identifying a suitable venue that can accommodate the required equipment storage and offer ample parking space.

Despite a sense of numbness, there were feelings of positivity and gratitude upon learning that my last treatment had reduced my PSA levels. However, I am also acutely aware that my days are numbered, which inspires me to try and make every moment count.

MY CLINICAL EXPERIENCE LEADING GROUP PROGRAMS

I worked in public health practice in Canada for ten years; for seven years I was part of the bladder clinic, in one of the biggest outpatient facilities in British Columbia, Canada. Because I started at the bladder clinic in its infancy, I was also responsible for setting up the physiotherapy program. From the start, I remember receiving a large number of post-prostatectomy referrals, patients who I had very little experience treating and supporting. Because of my lack of experience treating this population I started actively reviewing the literature to help me find the best approach to address their concerns. At the time men's health physiotherapy had very limited clinical resources—especially in the public sector—and pelvic floor muscle training (PFMT) for prostatectomy incontinence was not well supported in the literature.

Given that my waitlist was increasing, as well as the need to support this population, I decided to run a study to verify if a group physiotherapy program would be acceptable and feasible, and improve urinary outcomes for men post-prostatectomy. This study impacted my career, as I then realized how important it was to offer support to this population, especially by facilitating a positive environment for them to connect with each other, ask questions, and share emotions in a light-hearted way. I was also surprised how motivated they were to come to the sessions and how positive this experience was for them and for me. After the study ended and because of such positive outcomes, I developed a program for prostatectomy patients in the bladder clinic (before and after the surgery). They would be seen in a group format before they went on the physiotherapy waitlist in order to have the opportunity to receive information on the surgery and side-effects, PFMT, and bladder recovery, but mainly for them to interact with each other.

Many times, I noted the post-surgery patients helping and supporting the pre-surgery ones, and also the shift that happened in the atmosphere from the beginning to the end of the session. In the beginning of the session most of the men were worried, quiet, and not engaged, but afterwards they were all asking questions, sharing resources, and supporting each other. I felt that my role as a health professional was shifting from educating or lecturing on prostate cancer to supporting, caring, and facilitating interactions between prostate cancer patients in a safe and trusting environment. The interactions I had with these men and their families helped me become a better prostate cancer physiotherapist, for they promoted educational gains on prostate cancer and most importantly on prostate cancer patients' needs. These group sessions helped me realize the importance of socially supporting prostate cancer survivors, and the transformations that may occur to their wellbeing when they have meaningful connections with their peers.

SPIRITUALITY AND FAITH

Spirituality and religious practices may contribute to prostate cancer survivors' wellbeing and a sense of purpose. Spiritual institutions can also contribute to social support by providing a sense of community and belonging for individuals who share similar beliefs and values. Regular gatherings and events that are promoted by religious institutions may create a sense of social connectedness, allowing individuals to feel less isolated in their pursuit of a deeper connection to the divine.[37]

Spiritual insights can offer a sense of comfort, hope, and peace for individuals with cancer, allowing them to find meaning and purpose in their experiences and providing a framework for understanding the difficult emotions and challenges that come with a cancer diagnosis. Research has shown that individuals who have a strong sense of spirituality or religiosity may have better overall health outcomes, including lower rates of depression, anxiety, and substance abuse.[38] They may also have better coping mechanisms when facing illness or adversity.

---

37   (Jacobs, 2010)
38   (Lucchetti *et al.*, 2021)

Through spiritual practices and beliefs, men with prostate cancer may find a sense of resilience and inner strength, enabling them to maintain a positive outlook and continue to enjoy life despite the challenges posed by their illness and treatment.[39] Spirituality may also provide prostate cancer patients with a sense of clarity and guidance, allowing them to make decisions with greater confidence and ultimately reducing the likelihood of experiencing regret about their choices.[40] Moreover prostate cancer patients' sense of existential meaning and peace can be associated with improved physical, social, emotional, and functional wellbeing, and may be reverse-correlated with anxiety and depression.[41]

The recognition of spirituality in clinical practice and its incorporation into medical education have been driven by a growing body of scientific evidence that highlights the significant impact that spirituality can have on patient outcomes and the overall quality of care provided by healthcare professionals.[42] Therefore, physiotherapists and oncology clinicians' sensitivity to the role of religion, spirituality, and faith have the potential to not only improve prostate cancer survivors' quality of life but also promote greater satisfaction and engagement in their care.[43]

CONCLUSION

This chapter highlights the importance of social support in prostate cancer care. Social support can be received in many ways: through familial and partnership support, informal and formal peer support, prostate cancer group exercise programs, and religious/spiritual institutions. Recognizing the multidimensional nature of social support and promoting social engagement can play a vital role in improving health outcomes and overall wellbeing for prostate cancer patients, and as such, it is essential for physiotherapists and oncology clinicians to address these factors as part of their biopsychosocial care approach. Through group exercise programs, physiotherapists and oncology fitness professionals can provide a safe and supportive environment for prostate cancer patients to improve their physical health, while also offering opportunities for social interaction, emotional support, and a sense of community.

39   (Bergman *et al.*, 2011)
40   (Mollica *et al.*, 2017)
41   (Walker *et al.*, 2017)
42   (Lucchetti *et al.*, 2021)
43   (Bruce *et al.*, 2020)

REFERENCES

Baumeister, R.F., & Leary, M.R. (1995). The need to belong: Desire for interpersonal attachments as a fundamental human motivation. *Psychological Bulletin*, *117*(3), 497–529. https://doi.org/10.1037/0033-2909.117.3.497

Bergman, J., Fink, A., Kwan, L., Maliski, S., & Litwin, M.S. (2011). Spirituality and end-of-life care in disadvantaged men dying of prostate cancer. *World Journal of Urology*, *29*(1), 43–49. https://doi.org/10.1007/s00345-010-0610-y

Bruce, M.A., Bowie, J.V., Barge, H., Beech, B.M., LaVeist, T.A., Howard, D.L., & Thorpe, R.J. (2020). Religious coping and quality of life among Black and white men with prostate cancer. *Cancer Control: Journal of the Moffitt Cancer Center*, *27*(3), 1073274820936288. https://doi.org/10.1177/1073274820936288

Collaço, N., Wagland, R., Alexis, O., Gavin, A., Glaser, A., & Watson, E.K. (2019). The challenges on the family unit faced by younger couples affected by prostate cancer: A qualitative study. *Psycho-Oncology*, *28*(2), 329–335. https://doi.org/10.1002/pon.4944

Colloca, G., & Colloca, P. (2016). The effects of social support on health-related quality of life of patients with metastatic prostate cancer. *Journal of Cancer Education*, *31*(2), 244–252. https://doi.org/10.1007/s13187-015-0884-2

Costanzo, E.S., Sood, A.K., & Lutgendorf, S.K. (2011). Biobehavioral influences on cancer progression. *Immunology and Allergy Clinics*, *31*(1), 109–132. https://doi.org/10.1016/j.iac.2010.09.001

Cutrona, C.E., & Russell, D.W. (1990). Type of Social Support and Specific Stress: Toward a Theory of Optimal Matching. In B.R. Sarason, I.G. Sarason, & G.R. Pierce (eds), *Social Support: An Interactional View*. Hoboken, NJ: John Wiley & Sons.

Cuypers, M., Lamers, R.E.D., Kil, P.J.M., Cornel, E.B., van de Poll-Franse, L.V., & de Vries, M. (2018). The impact of prostate cancer diagnosis and treatment decision-making on health-related quality of life before treatment onset. *Supportive Care in Cancer*, *26*(4), 1297–1304. https://doi.org/10.1007/s00520-017-3953-8

Dunn, J., Ralph, N., Green, A., Frydenberg, M., & Chambers, S.K. (2020). Contemporary consumer perspectives on prostate cancer survivorship: Fifty voices. *Psycho-Oncology*, *29*(3), 557–563. https://doi.org/10.1002/pon.5306

Fernandez-Portero, C., Amian, J.G., Alarcón, D., Arenilla Villalba, M.J., & Sánchez-Medina, J.A. (2023). The effect of social relationships on the well-being and happiness of older adults living alone or with relatives. *Healthcare*, *11*(2), 222. https://doi.org/10.3390/healthcare11020222

Garrett, B.M., Oliffe, J.L., Bottorff, J.L., McKenzie, M., Han, C.S., & Ogrodniczuk, J.S. (2014). The value of prostate cancer support groups: A pilot study of primary physicians' perspectives. *BMC Family Practice*, *15*, 56. https://doi.org/10.1186/1471-2296-15-56

Jacobs, C. (2010). Exploring religion and spirituality in clinical practice. *Smith College Studies in Social Work*, *80*(2–3), 98–120. https://doi.org/10.1080/00377317.2010.486358

Jan, M., Bonn, S.E., Sjölander, A., Wiklund, F., *et al.* (2016). The roles of stress and social support in prostate cancer mortality. *Scandinavian Journal of Urology*, *50*(1), 47–55. https://doi.org/10.3109/21681805.2015.1079796

Jones, M., & Pietilä, I. (2020). Expertise, advocacy and activism: A qualitative study on the activities of prostate cancer peer support workers. *Health (London, England: 1997)*, *24*(1), 21–37. https://doi.org/10.1177/1363459318785711

Lazarus, R.S., & Folkman, S. (1984). *Stress, Appraisal, and Coping*. New York: Springer Publishing Company.

Lee, M., Nielsen, T., & Ma, J. (2020). Danish experiences of "togetherness" and its implications for multicultural education. *Multicultural Education Review*, *12*(1), 1–3. https://doi.org/10.1080/2005615X.2020.1720291

Lucchetti, G., Koenig, H.G., & Lucchetti, A.L.G. (2021). Spirituality, religiousness, and mental health: A review of the current scientific evidence. *World Journal of Clinical Cases*, *9*(26), 7620–7631. https://doi.org/10.12998/wjcc.v9.i26.7620

Martire, L.M., Lustig, A.P., Schulz, R., Miller, G.E., & Helgeson, V.S. (2004). Is it beneficial to involve a family member? A meta-analysis of psychosocial interventions for chronic illness. *Health Psychology: Official Journal of the Division of Health Psychology, American Psychological Association, 23*(6), 599–611. https://doi.org/10.1037/0278-6133.23.6.599

Mead, S., Hilton, D., & Curtis, L. (2001). Peer support: A theoretical perspective. *Psychiatric Rehabilitation Journal, 25*(2), 134–141. https://doi.org/10.1037/h0095032

Mollica, M.A., Underwood, W., Ill, Homish, G.G., Homish, D.L., & Orom, H. (2017). Spirituality is associated with less treatment regret in men with localized prostate cancer. *Psycho-Oncology, 26*(11), 1839–1845. https://doi.org/10.1002/pon.4248

Mukwato, K.P., Mweemba, P., Makukula, M.K., & Makoleka, M.M. (2010). Stress and coping mechanisms among breast cancer patients and family caregivers: A review of literature. *Medical Journal of Zambia, 37*(1), Article 1. https://doi.org/10.4314/mjz.v37i1

Paltiel, H., Solvoll, E., Loge, J.H., Kaasa, S., & Oldervoll, L. (2009). "The healthy me appears": Palliative cancer patients' experiences of participation in a physical group exercise program. *Palliative & Supportive Care, 7*(4), 459–467. https://doi.org/10.1017/S1478951509990460

Schlichthorst, M., Ozols, I., Reifels, L., & Morgan, A. (2020). Lived experience peer support programs for suicide prevention: A systematic scoping review. *International Journal of Mental Health Systems, 14*. https://doi.org/10.1186/s13033-020-00396-1

Varner, S., Lloyd, G., Ranby, K.W., Callan, S., Robertson, C., & Lipkus, I.M. (2019). Illness uncertainty, partner support, and quality of life: A dyadic longitudinal investigation of couples facing prostate cancer. *Psycho-Oncology, 28*(11), 2188–2194. https://doi.org/10.1002/pon.5205

Vyas, N., Brunckhorst, O., Fox, L., Van Hemelrijck, M., *et al.* (2022). Undergoing radical treatment for prostate cancer and its impact on wellbeing: A qualitative study exploring men's experiences. *PLoS One, 17*(12), e0279250. https://doi.org/10.1371/journal.pone.0279250

Walker, S.J., Chen, Y., Paik, K., Mirly, B., Thomas, C.R., Jr, & Hung, A.Y. (2017). The relationships between spiritual well-being, quality of life, and psychological factors before radiotherapy for prostate cancer. *Journal of Religion and Health, 56*(5), 1846–1855. https://doi.org/10.1007/s10943-016-0352-2

Wiking, M. (2016). *The Little Book of Hygge: The Danish Way to Live Well.* New York: Penguin Random House.

World Happiness Report (n.d.). Trust and social connections in times of crisis. Retrieved March 20, 2023, from https://worldhappiness.report/ed/2023/world-happiness-trust-and-social-connections-in-times-of-crisis

Zhang, A.Y., Strauss, G.J., & Siminoff, L.A. (2007). Effects of combined pelvic floor muscle exercise and a support group on urinary incontinence and quality of life of postprostatectomy patients. *Oncology Nursing Forum, 34*(1), 47–53. https://doi.org/10.1188/07.ONF.47-53

Zhao, X., Sun, M., & Yang, Y. (2021). Effects of social support, hope and resilience on depressive symptoms within 18 months after diagnosis of prostate cancer. *Health and Quality of Life Outcomes, 19*(1), 15. https://doi.org/10.1186/s12955-020-01660-1

CHAPTER 12

Summary and Final Thoughts

Prostate cancer is a very prominent disease in the world, affecting millions of men and their families.[1] The diagnosis of prostate cancer can be a life-altering event, significantly impacting patients' quality of life and overall wellbeing. Although treatment can be highly effective for localized prostate cancer, most of the men diagnosed with this disease can find that it has detrimental consequences for their physical and emotional state. Side-effects of treatment such as urinary incontinence and sexual dysfunctions may profoundly affect men's self-esteem and relationships. Additionally, the emotional toll of the diagnosis and treatment can be significant, leading to anxiety, depression, and other mental health concerns.[2]

This book introduced a biopsychosocial humanistic approach in addressing prostate cancer survivorship, with a focus on promoting a strong therapeutic alliance between patients and clinicians. Adopting a patient-centered approach that emphasizes mutual understanding, respect, and cultural sensitivity can help clinicians establish a strong bond with their prostate cancer patients, ultimately leading to the development of more personalized and effective treatment plans. This approach may improve treatment efficacy by addressing the unique needs and concerns of each patient, resulting in a more positive and empowering healthcare experience. Compassionate care and compassion training may help physiotherapists and oncology clinicians improve emotional resilience and professional satisfaction, allowing them to provide optimal client-focused care.

As a part of comprehensive care for prostate cancer, evidence is increasing to support the inclusion of exercise therapy and pelvic floor rehabilitation. These treatments can assist in managing the side-effects of cancer and treatments, which include urinary incontinence, erectile dysfunction, fatigue, and emotional distress. In fact, incorporating pelvic floor rehabilitation before radical prostatectomy surgery has been found to be beneficial in improving urinary incontinence after surgery. Furthermore, physiotherapy visits prior to prostate cancer treatments can be valuable in mitigating the effects of

---

1   (DeSantis et al., 2014)
2   (Sennfält et al., 2004)

treatment. These visits can help identify areas that may require targeted exercises, other interventions, or referrals to other practitioners, such as the patient's pelvic floor muscles and mental health status. An integrated care approach that includes pelvic floor rehabilitation, exercise therapy, pressure management, bladder training, emotional support, and/or the use of passive devices may be needed in improving urinary outcomes and reducing the mental health risks faced by prostate cancer patients experiencing urinary incontinence.

Although there is evidence to support the effectiveness of pelvic floor rehabilitation in improving urinary incontinence in prostate cancer survivors who have undergone surgery, research on its efficacy for improving urinary function in individuals who have undergone other treatments such as radiation and hormonal therapy is still limited. In addition, there is limited data on the effects of pelvic floor rehabilitation and other conservative methods for improving bowel and sexual function after prostate cancer treatments. Given the importance of addressing these symptoms to enhance survivors' quality of life, and the potential for pelvic floor rehabilitation and other lower-cost conservative treatments to improve urinary, bowel, and sexual function, further research is needed to gain a more comprehensive understanding of the benefits of these treatments for a wider range of individuals with prostate cancer. Continued research in this area is particularly important given the potential for pelvic floor rehabilitation and other conservative treatments to provide effective symptom management with fewer side-effects than more invasive treatment options. As such, it may be critical for further investigation into the potential benefits of pelvic floor rehabilitation and other conservative treatments in prostate cancer survivors, in order to optimize care and improve outcomes.

Exercise is a critical therapy for improving function, reducing pain, enhancing quality of life, and mitigating the negative effects of cancer.[3, 4, 5] However, despite its numerous benefits, there is a pressing need to provide more support to prostate cancer survivors in order to increase their engagement in the recommended levels of exercise.[6] Identifying barriers to the promotion of exercise therapy in prostate cancer care is an important step in increasing the number of prostate cancer survivors who engage in the recommended amount of exercise. Some possible barriers that may prevent survivors from participating in exercise therapy include lack of knowledge or awareness of the benefits of exercise, lack of motivation or interest, physical limitations or discomfort, financial barriers, lack of access to exercise facilities or programs, and competing demands on their time. Addressing these

---

3   (Seguin & Nelson, 2003)
4   (Carrasco *et al.*, 2020)
5   (Wollesen *et al.*, 2017)
6   (Cormie *et al.*, 2015)

barriers may require a multi-faceted approach, such as providing educational materials and resources on the benefits of exercise, offering tailored exercise programs that accommodate survivors' physical limitations or discomfort, providing financial assistance or incentives, improving access to exercise facilities or programs, and offering support or encouragement to survivors to help them overcome competing demands on their time. Group exercise programs specifically designed for prostate cancer survivors can provide an additional incentive for them to engage in physical activity, while also offering the benefit of social support. Additionally, physiotherapists, physicians, and oncology clinicians can play a key role in promoting exercise therapy by discussing the benefits of exercise with their patients, prescribing exercise as part of their treatment plan, and monitoring their progress and adherence to the exercise regimen.

This book also emphasized the significance of adequately equipping physiotherapists and healthcare professionals in oncology with the knowledge of identifying signs and symptoms of mental health issues, as well as the process of providing appropriate support and resources for those in need. Psychological screening and psychosocial interventions can significantly benefit prostate cancer survivors, who are at higher risk of experiencing mental distress that may negatively impact their symptoms, prognosis, and quality of life.[7]

Prostate cancer can greatly affect male sexual wellbeing, underscoring the importance of raising awareness early in the journey of prostate cancer patients. Implementing penile rehabilitation, providing intimacy support, and involving partners in sexual discussions can enhance sexual outcomes and contribute to an improved overall cancer experience for prostate cancer patients.

Social support and integration play a valuable role in improving prostate cancer patients' health outcomes, sense of belonging, and overall wellbeing.[8] Providing social support to prostate cancer survivors, which includes familial and partner support, informal and formal peer support, group exercise programs, and involvement with religious or spiritual institutions, may substantially impact their treatment outcomes. Increased social support has been linked to improved cancer outlook, resilience, and self-efficacy.[9] Physiotherapists and other health professionals can facilitate social support for prostate cancer patients in various ways. For instance, they can encourage patients to join local support groups and provide them with relevant information. Additionally, involving family members and partners in sessions, using technology to facilitate engagement in social media platforms and online support groups, partnering with religious or spiritual institutions, incorporating social activities into treatment plans, and organizing group

7   (Dinesh *et al.*, 2021)
8   (Costanzo *et al.*, 2011)
9   (Cuypers *et al.*, 2018)

activities or programs are other effective ways to increase social support for prostate cancer patients.

In conclusion, prostate cancer care can be integrative, motivational, culturally adaptive, personal, attentive, compassionate, approachable, responsible, and supportive. Integrating a humanistic biopsychosocial approach into physiotherapy and oncology care can potentially improve the outcomes and satisfaction of prostate cancer care for patients, their families, and healthcare providers.

REFERENCES

Carrasco, C., Tomas-Carus, P., Bravo, J., Pereira, C., & Mendes, F. (2020). Understanding fall risk factors in community-dwelling older adults: A cross-sectional study. *International Journal of Older People Nursing, 15*(1). https://doi.org/10.1111/opn.12294

Cormie, P., Turner, B., Kaczmarek, E., Drake, D., & Chambers, S.K. (2015). A qualitative exploration of the experience of men with prostate cancer involved in supervised exercise programs. *Oncology Nursing Forum, 42*(1), 24–32. https://doi.org/10.1188/15.ONF.24-32

Costanzo, E.S., Sood, A.K., & Lutgendorf, S.K. (2011). Biobehavioral influences on cancer progression. *Immunology and Allergy Clinics, 31*(1), 109–132. https://doi.org/10.1016/j.iac.2010.09.001

Cuypers, M., Lamers, R.E.D., Kil, P.J.M., Cornel, E.B., van de Poll-Franse, L.V., & de Vries, M. (2018). The impact of prostate cancer diagnosis and treatment decision-making on health-related quality of life before treatment onset. *Supportive Care in Cancer, 26*(4), 1297–1304. https://doi.org/10.1007/s00520-017-3953-8

DeSantis, C.E., Lin, C.C., Mariotto, A.B., Siegel, R.L., *et al.* (2014). Cancer treatment and survivorship statistics, 2014. *CA: A Cancer Journal for Clinicians, 64*(4), 252–271. https://doi.org/10.3322/caac.21235

Dinesh, A.A., Helena Pagani Soares Pinto, S., Brunckhorst, O., Dasgupta, P., & Ahmed, K. (2021). Anxiety, depression and urological cancer outcomes: A systematic review. *Urologic Oncology: Seminars and Original Investigations, 39*(12), 816–828. https://doi.org/10.1016/j.urolonc.2021.08.003

Seguin, R., & Nelson, M.E. (2003). The benefits of strength training for older adults. *American Journal of Preventive Medicine, 25*(3 Suppl. 2), 141–149. https://doi.org/10.1016/s0749-3797(03)00177-6

Sennfält, K., Carlsson, P., Sandblom, G., & Varenhorst, E. (2004). The estimated economic value of the welfare loss due to prostate cancer pain in a defined population. *Acta Oncologica (Stockholm, Sweden), 43*(3), 290–296. https://doi.org/10.1080/02841860410028411

Wollesen, B., Mattes, K., Schulz, S., Bischoff, L.L., Seydell, L., Bell, J.W., & von Duvillard, S.P. (2017). Effects of dual-task management and resistance training on gait performance in older individuals: A randomized controlled trial. *Frontiers in Aging Neuroscience, 19*, 415. https://doi.org/10.3389/fnagi.2017.00415

APPENDICES

All handouts and activities marked with a ✔ can be photocopied or downloaded from http://www.jkp.com/catalogue/book/9781839975561

Appendix 1: Biopsychosocial History Taking

✓

BIOPSYCHOSOCIAL HISTORY TAKING	
<u>Main symptoms or concerns</u>	Date of prostate cancer diagnosis: Date of beginning and ending treatment: Gleason score: PSA present: PSA before treatment: Name of urologist/oncologist:
<u>Emotional status and sleep</u>	<u>Questionnaires</u> ICIQ-SF: NCCN DT and PL: Other:
<u>Activity history</u> Current activity participation/exercise: Activities avoided due to symptoms: Activity goals:	
<u>Social history</u> Occupation: Relationship: Family: Hobbies:	<u>Social support</u> ized <u>Spiritual practices</u>
<u>Past medical history</u>	<u>Medications</u>

✓

BIOPSYCHOSOCIAL HISTORY TAKING cont.

Investigations

(Urodynamics, cystoscopy, CT-scan, others):

Urinary symptoms

Amount of drinks:

Amount of caffeinated or alcoholic drinks:

Frequency of voids:

Amount of urine:

Amount of leakage:

Difficulties at starting stream:

Blood in the urine:

Urgency:

Dribbling urination:

Holding time:

Nocturia:

Number of pads and pads volume:

Skin condition:

Bowel history

Continence:

Frequency:

Stool quality:

Diet, fiber intake:

Sexual history

Sexual symptoms:

Previous symptoms prior to treatments:

Partner:

History of trauma, or adverse childhood experiences:

Sexual goals:

Meaningful goals

Long-term:

Short-term:

Other comments

Appendix 2: Bladder and Bowel Diary

The bladder and bowel diary is a tool that provides valuable information about your fluid intake, urination habits, and bladder leaks, as well as bowel movements. This data may help you better understand your condition and quantify your changes. Here are some guidelines for using the bladder and bowel diary:

- Record the time of day you drink, urinate, or experience leaks in the "time" column, including nighttime.
- Note the type and quantity of fluid you drink in the "drink" column, using units such as ml, ounces, or cups.
- When emptying your bladder, measure the amount of urine in a container and record it in the "urine amount" column. If you cannot measure it, estimate the amount as small, medium, or large.
- If you experience bladder leaks, indicate the amount (small, medium, or large) in the "leak" column, and identify the potential cause (e.g., cough, sudden movement). If the cause was an urge, rate its strength on a scale of 1 to 5.
- For bowel movements, describe the type of stool using the legend provided. If you leak stool, record the type, amount, and possible trigger, as well as the strength of the urge (0 to 5).
- Repeat this process for three consecutive days.

Bowel type	Description
Type 1	Hard pellets
Type 2	Formed and hard
Type 3	Formed and soft
Type 4	Toothpaste like
Type 5	Liquid

✓ 24-HOUR BLADDER AND BOWEL DIARY

Name: _____   Date: _____   Day #1 #2 #3

Time	Amount/type of drink	Urine amount	Stool type (1 to 5)	Leaking		Strong urge	
				Urine	Stool	Urine	Stool

Number of pads used in 24 hours: _____

24-HOUR PAD TEST

The 24-hour pad test is a highly dependable way to monitor urine leakage and track your progress. This test involves weighing the pads used in a 24-hour period to determine the amount of urine leakage in grams. Here are the steps to follow:

Step 1: Place frequently used pads in a ziplock bag, enough for a 24-hour period.

Step 2: Weigh the ziplock bag containing the unused pads using a kitchen scale and record the weight in grams. This will be your dry pads weight (DP).

Step 3: On the day of the test, use the pads from the ziplock bag for the entire 24-hour period, without discarding any used pads or their plastic wrapping.

Step 4: At the end of the 24 hours, weigh the same ziplock bag with both the used pads and the unused pads with their wrappings. This will be the used (wet) pads weight (WP).

Step 5: Calculate the amount of urine leaked in grams by subtracting the weight of the ziplock bag containing only the dry pads from the weight measurement of the bag containing both the used (wet) and unused pads with their wrappings (WP–DP). This difference will give you the weight of the urine leaked.

Step 6: Repeat this process every 1–2 months.

✓ 24-HOUR PAD TEST TABLE

Date	Dry pads' weight (g)	Wet pads' weight (g)	Total loss of urine (g)

Subject Index

Author Index